AF594134

TESTICULAR TUMORS

TESTICULAR TUMORS

Robert H. Young, MD, MRCPath
Associate Pathologist
Massachusetts General Hospital, Boston
Associate Professor of Pathology
Harvard Medical School, Boston

Robert E. Scully, MD
Pathologist
Massachusetts General Hospital, Boston
Professor of Pathology
Harvard Medical School, Boston

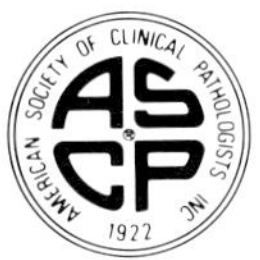

ASCP Press
American Society of Clinical Pathologists
Chicago

Cover: Large cell calcifying Sertoli cell tumor (see Figure 5.25).

Library of Congress Cataloging-in-Publication Data

Young, Robert H. (Robert Henry), 1950–
Testicular tumors / Robert H. Young, Robert E. Scully.
Includes bibliographical references.
ISBN 0-89189-295-8
1. Testis—Tumors—Histopathology—Atlases. I. Scully, Robert E. (Robert Edward), 1921– . II. Title.
[DNLM: 1. Testicular Neoplasms—atlases. WJ 17 Y75a]
RC280.T4Y68 1990
616.99'263—dc20
DNLM/DLC/
for Library of Congress 90–18
CIP

Printed in the United States of America.

94 93 92 91 90 5 4 3 2 1

Contents

Preface IX

1 **Classification and Staging 1**
References 7

2 **Germ Cell Tumors: Seminomas 9**
Seminoma 9
Spermatocytic Seminoma 12
References 33

3 **Germ Cell Tumors: Nonseminomatous Tumors, Occult Tumors, Effects of Chemotherapy 37**
Embryonal Carcinoma 37
Yolk Sac Tumor (Endodermal Sinus Tumor) 38
Choriocarcinoma 40
Polyembryoma 41
Teratoma 41
Carcinoid Tumor 42
Primitive Neuroectodermal Tumor 43
Tumors of More Than One Histological Type (Mixed Germ Cell Tumors) 44
Occult Testicular Germ Cell Tumors 46
Germ Cell Tumors After Chemotherapy 47
References 84

4 Intratubular Germ Cell Neoplasia 89

Intratubular Germ Cell Neoplasia, Unclassified 89
Intratubular Seminoma 92
Intratubular Embryonal Carcinoma 92
Other Forms of Intratubular Germ Cell Neoplasia 93
References 99

5 Sex Cord–Stromal Tumors 101

Leydig Cell Tumors 101
Sertoli Cell Tumors 104
Granulosa Cell Tumors 106
Sex Cord–Stromal Tumors, Unclassified 108
References 135

6 Tumors and Tumorlike Lesions in Intersexual Disorders 137

Mixed Gonadal Dysgenesis 137
True Hermaphroditism 139
Androgen Insensitivity Syndrome 140
References 150

7 Hematopoietic and Metastatic Tumors 151

Malignant Lymphoma 151
Multiple Myeloma and Plasmacytoma 152
Leukemia 153
Metastatic Tumors 153
References 161

8 Miscellaneous Tumors Including Adnexal Tumors 163

Adenomatoid Tumor 163
Malignant Mesothelioma 164
Tumors of Ovarian Epithelial Types 164
Tumors of the Rete Testis 165
Papillary Cystadenoma and Carcinoma of the Epididymis 166
Retinal Anlage Tumor 167
Soft Tissue Tumors 167
References 186

9 Nonneoplastic Lesions 189
Adrenocortical Rests 189
Testicular 'Tumors' of the Androgenital Syndrome 189
Cysts 191
Cystic Dysplasia 191
Nodular Precocious Maturation 192
Orchitis 192
Malakoplakia 194
Fibromatous Periorchitis (Fibrous Pseudotumor) (Nodular Periorchitis) 195
Cholesterol Granuloma and Calcification of Tunica Vaginalis 196
Sclerosing Lipogranuloma 196
Splenic-Gonadal Fusion 196
Infarcts and Hematomas 197
Sperm Granuloma of the Epididymis and Vas Deferens 197
References 222

Index 225

Preface

Testicular tumors are of great interest to both the clinician and the pathologist, to the clinician because they are almost always malignant and most of them are highly responsive to therapy, and to the pathologist because almost all of them are of germ cell origin, with a potential for differentiation in many directions. This atlas and text will explore the morphologic features of these tumors with emphasis on variations in their appearance and their differential diagnosis. Clinical aspects that are of major interest to the pathologist will also be presented.

Despite the complex pathology of testicular tumors and related lesions, a relatively small number of texts has been devoted to them over the years. In the past decade conventional light microscopic studies have elucidated the features of several new subtypes of testicular tumor and the application of immunohistochemistry to the study of testicular neoplasms is another recent development. These facts, as well as the continuing diagnostic challenge that these tumors provide, should make this text and atlas timely from the viewpoint of the practicing pathologist. Although immunohistochemical staining has increased our understanding of testicular tumors and in occasional cases has been helpful diagnostically, careful examination of well-prepared specimens stained in the conventional manner remains the cornerstone of accurate pathologic diagnosis; accordingly, the majority of the illustrations of microscopic sections are of preparations stained by hematoxylin and eosin.

Although many of the specimens illustrated are from our institution, a significant number, including a disproportionate number of the unusual lesions, are of cases seen in consultation and we are grateful to the numerous pathologists who have shared this material with us. We are also grateful to Mr Stephen Conley and Ms Michelle Forrestall for their invaluable help in taking most of the photographs.

1 Classification and Staging

A classification of testicular tumors and tumorlike lesions similar to that of the World Health Organization[1] is presented in Table 1.1.

Table 1.1
Histological Classification of Testicular Tumors

Germ Cell Tumors
- Tumors of One Histological Type
  - Seminoma
    - Variant: seminoma with syncytiotrophoblast cells
  - Spermatocytic seminoma
  - Embryonal carcinoma
  - Yolk sac tumor (endodermal sinus tumor)
  - Choriocarcinoma
  - Polyembryoma
  - Teratoma
    - Mature
    - Immature
    - Monodermal and highly specialized
      - Carcinoid
      - Primitive neuroectodermal tumors
      - Others
    - With malignant transformation
- Tumors of More Than One Histological Type
  - Embryonal carcinoma and teratoma (teratocarcinoma)
  - Other combinations (specify)
- Intratubular Germ Cell Neoplasia

(Continued.)

Table 1.1
Continued.

Sex Cord–Stromal Tumors

- Pure forms
  - Leydig cell tumor
  - Sertoli cell tumor
    - Variants
    - Large-cell calcifying
    - Lipid-rich
  - Granulosa cell tumor
    - Adult
    - Juvenile
- Mixed forms (specify)
- Unclassified

Tumors Containing Germ Cells and Sex Cord–Stromal Elements

- Gonadoblastoma
- Unclassified

Tumors and Tumorlike Lesions of Androgen Insensitivity Syndrome

- Hamartomas
- Sertoli cell adenoma
- Leydig cell tumor
- Malignant sex cord tumor
- Germ cell tumors
- Adnexal cysts

Tumors of Hematopoietic System

Secondary Tumors

Miscellaneous Tumors Including Adnexal Tumors

- Adenomatoid tumor
- Mesothelioma
- Tumors of ovarian epithelial types
- Adenoma of rete testis
- Carcinoma of rete testis
- Cystadenoma of epididymis
- Carcinoma of epididymis
- Melanotic neuroectodermal tumor (retinal anlage tumor)
- Soft tissue tumors

Unclassified Tumors

Tumorlike Lesions

- Adrenal rest
- 'Tumor' of the adrenogenital syndrome

(Continued.)

Table 1.1
Continued.

- Cysts
  - Epidermoid
  - Others
- Cystic dysplasia
- Nodular precocious maturation
- Orchitis
  - Infectious
  - Granulomatous, idiopathic
  - Malakoplakia
- Fibromatous periorchitis
- Cholesterol granuloma
- Lipogranuloma
- Splenic-gonadal fusion
- Infarct
- Hematoma
- Sperm granuloma
- Others

The staging of testicular germ cell tumors, which is of great importance in the determination of prognosis and therapy, requires not only careful clinical, radiologic, and laboratory investigation, but also meticulous gross and microscopic examination of the excised specimens. The rules for tumor, lymph node, metastasis (TNM) staging of testicular tumors are presented below in Table 1.2.[2] For clinical staging, clinical examination and radical orchiectomy are required. For pathologic staging, histologic evaluation of the radical orchiectomy specimen must be used for the pT stage. The specimens from a defined node-bearing area (ie, retroperitoneal node dissection) must be used for the pN stage. Histologic verification is required.

When the specimen is received in the laboratory, the dimensions, extent, and other gross features of the tumor should be described and thin sections should be taken promptly and fixed adequately. At least one section per centimeter of greatest diameter of the tumor is optimal. The sections should include the adjacent testicular parenchyma, the rete testis, and the portion of tunica albuginea closest to the neoplasm. All areas with differing gross features must be sampled. Sections of the epididymis, lower spermatic cord, spermatic cord resection margin, and any area suggestive of tumor elsewhere in the cord should also be obtained. An adequate microscopic description includes mention of the extent of the neoplasm, identification of all of its subtypes, and a comment on the presence or absence of intratubular germ cell neoplasia in the adjacent testis. Vascular space

Table 1.2
TNM Staging of Testicular Cancer

Extent of Primary Tumor (T)

TX	Primary tumor cannot be assessed (in the absence of radical orchiectomy, TX is used)
T0	Histologic scar or no evidence of primary tumor
Tis	Intratubular tumor: preinvasive cancer
T1	Tumor limited to testis, including rete testis
T2	Tumor invades beyond tunica albuginea or into epididymis
T3	Tumor invades spermatic cord
T4	Tumor invades scrotum

Regional Lymph Nodes (N)

NX	Regional lymph nodes cannot be assessed
N0	No regional lymph node metastasis
N1	Metastasis in a single lymph node, 2 cm or less in greatest dimension
N2	Metastasis in a single lymph node, more than 2 cm, but not more than 5 cm in greatest dimension, or multiple lymph nodes, none more than 5 cm in greatest dimension
N3	Metastasis in a lymph node more than 5 cm in greatest dimension

Distant Metastasis (M)

MX	Presence of distant metastasis cannot be assessed
M0	No distant metastasis
M1	Distant metastasis

Stage Grouping

Stage 0	Tis	N0	M0
Stage I	T1	N0	M0
	T2	N0	M0
Stage II	T3	N0	M0
	T4	N0	M0
Stage III	Any T	N1	M0
Stage IV	Any T	N2, N3	M0
	Any T	Any N	M1

invasion (Figure 1.1) has proved to be an important indicator of prognosis[3–6] and is one of a number of factors that may determine whether a patient with a Stage I tumor will receive additional therapy or will be followed expectantly.[7–9] Therefore, a comment on the presence or absence of this feature should also be included in the pathology report. Determination of vascular space invasion may be more difficult in the testis than in other organs and tissues. Very cellular tumors such as seminoma and embryonal carcinoma may be "buttered" into gaping vessels by the sectioning knife (Figure 1.2).

This artifactual pseudoinvasion is characterized by the presence of aggregates of loosely arranged cells that do not conform to the shapes of the vascular lumina. In addition, some forms of intratubular neoplasia may simulate venous invasion. The location of the structure containing the neoplastic cells and the differing patterns of elastic tissue in vein walls and the walls of sclerotic tubules may aid in the differential diagnosis of venous and intratubular neoplasia. The use of immunohistochemical staining of endothelial cells for factor VIII–related antigen and *Ulex europaeus* 1 lectin antigens, particularly the latter,[10] may also be helpful in establishing the vascular nature of a space that contains tumor.

The relative amounts of the various components of mixed germ cell tumors should also be estimated, as some investigators have found component quantitation, particularly the amount of embryonal carcinoma,[6,9] to have prognostic significance. Finally, if unsampled tumor remains in the specimen, it is desirable to retain it until it becomes evident that the clinical course of the patient is consistent with the pathological diagnosis.

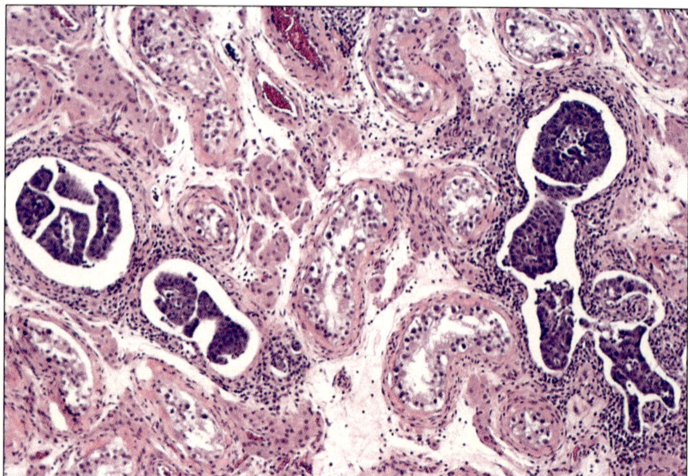

Figure 1.1 Vascular invasion by embryonal carcinoma. Note that the intravascular tumor conforms to the shapes of the vessels.

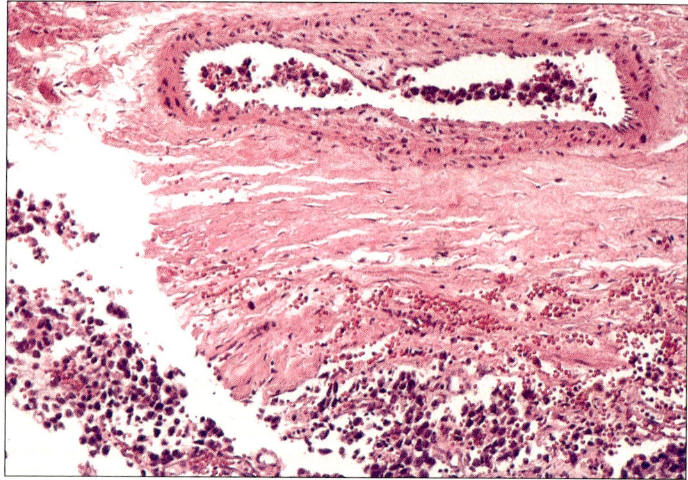

Figure 1.2 Artifactual presence of seminoma cells within a vessel and along the edge of the section. Note that the intravascular tumor does not conform to the shape of the vessel and is composed of dispersed degenerating cells.

References

1. Mostofi FK, Sobin LH. Histological typing of tumours of the testis. *International Histological Classification of Tumours,* No. 16. Geneva, World Health Organization, 1977.
2. *Manual for Staging of Cancer, American Joint Committee on Cancer, ed 3.* Beahrs OH, Henson DE, Hutter RVP, eds. Philadelphia, JB Lippincott Co, 1988, pp 184–185.
3. Fujime M, Chang, H, Lin C-W, Prout GR. Correlation of vascular invasion and metastasis in germ cell tumors of testis: A preliminary report. *J Urol* 131:1237–1241, 1984.
4. Freedman LS, Parkinson, MC, Jones WG, et al. Histopathology in the prediction of relapse of patients with stage I testicular teratoma treated by orchiectomy alone. *Lancet* 2:294–298, 1987.
5. Hoskin P, Dilly S, Easton D, Horwich A, Hendry W, Peckham MJ. Prognostic factors in stage I non-seminomatous germ-cell testicular tumours managed by orchiectomy and surveillance: Implications for adjuvant chemotherapy. *J Clin Oncol* 4:1031-1036, 1986.
6. Javadpour N, Young JD. Prognostic factors in nonseminomatous testicular cancer. *J Urol* 135:497-499, 1986.
7. Fung CY, Garnick MB. Clinical stage I carcinoma of the testis: A review. *J Clin Oncol* 6:734–750, 1988.
8. Raghavan D, Vogelzang NJ, Bosl GJ, Nochomovitz LE, Rosai J, et al. Tumor classification and size in germ-cell testicular cancer: Influence on the occurrence of metastases. *Cancer* 50:1591–1595, 1982.
9. Dunphy CH, Ayala, AG, Swanson DA, Ro JY, Logothetis C. Clinical stage I nonseminomatous and mixed germ cell tumors of the testis: A clinico-pathologic study of 93 patients on a surveillance protocol after orchiectomy alone. *Cancer* 62:1202–1206, 1988.
10. Little D, Said JW, Siegel RJ, Fealy M, Fishbein MC. Endothelial cell markers in vascular neoplasms: An immunohistochemical study comparing factor VIII-related antigen, blood group specific antigens, 6-keto-PGF1 alpha, and *Ulex europaeus* 1 lectin. *J Pathol* 149:89–95, 1986.

Germ Cell Tumors: Seminomas 2

Germ cell tumors account for over 90% of testicular tumors[1–3] and for slightly over 1% of all cancers in males.[4] If leukemia and lymphoma are excluded, these tumors are the most frequent form of cancer in men between 15 and 34 years of age.[5] They arise from five to ten times more frequently in cryptorchid than in descended testes.[1,2,6–8] The increased frequency of germ cell tumors in cryptorchid testes persists after orchidopexy; a descended testis contralateral to a cryptorchid testis also has an enhanced susceptibility to germ cell neoplasia. There are striking differences worldwide in the incidence of testicular germ cell tumors, with the highest incidence in Denmark, Norway, and New Zealand, and the lowest in Finland, the Orient, black Africa, and Puerto Rico.[9] The incidence is much lower in blacks than in whites in the United States.[9] The causes of these striking variations are unknown.

Seminoma

Seminomas, which account for approximately 50% of testicular germ cell tumors,[10] are composed of primitive-appearing germ cells that typically fail to differentiate.[11–14] Over 95% of these tumors are typical, or "classic," seminomas composed of cells that resemble the primordial germ cells of the embryo. The designation "anaplastic seminoma" has been used for seminomas with high mitotic counts.[15,16] There has been significant interobserver and intraobserver variation in mitotic counting in seminomas,[17,18] however, and although seminomas with high mitotic rates appear to present at a higher stage than tumors with fewer mitotic figures,[16] there is no convincing evidence that so-called anaplastic seminomas, stage for stage, have a worse prognosis than typical seminomas.[15] Therefore, the designation anaplastic is not warranted except for investigative purposes at the present time. About 10% of seminomas contain varying numbers of syncytiotrophoblast cells, which may secrete measurable quantities of chorionic gonadotropin (hCG) into the serum.[19–21] The spermatocytic seminoma has clinical and pathological features that are distinct from those of the typical seminoma and will be discussed separately.

Typical seminomas reach their peak age incidence between 35 and 45 years,[10] are relatively uncommon in men over 50 years of age, and are very rare in children.[22] The great majority of the patients present because of testicular swelling,[23] but gynecomastia is an initial manifestation in approximately 1% of the cases,[24] and occasionally patients present with symptoms related to tumor at a metastatic site. Very rarely, exophthalmos, apparently on a paraendocrine basis, is a presenting feature.[25,26] Seminomas are bilateral, usually metachronously, in only 2% to 5% of the cases, but account for the majority of bilateral germ cell tumors.[27–30] Approximately 8% of seminomas occur in undescended testes[2] or testes that had been cryptorchid but were surgically placed in the scrotum. The testis is usually enlarged by a seminoma, but in approximately 10% to 15% of the cases, it is normal in size or even atrophic.[1]

Gross examination typically reveals a well-circumscribed mass with a uniform, lobulated, white, cream-colored, or pink sectioned surface (Figure 2.1). The neoplastic tissue may be soft or firm, depending on the relative amounts of tumor cells and fibrous stroma (Figure 2.2). Some tumors contain sharply demarcated foci of caseationlike necrosis; occasionally, large areas of necrosis (Figure 2.3), hemorrhage, or both are encountered. Rare tumors are red (Figure 2.4), and small punctate foci of hemorrhage, which may indicate the presence of syncytiotrophoblast giant cells, are occasionally seen.[31] The finding of such atypical gross features warrants more thorough sampling than usual to exclude the presence of another form of germ cell tumor such as embryonal carcinoma or choriocarcinoma. Most tumors are confined to the testis, but extension to the epididymis or spermatic cord is seen in approximately 8% of the cases.[1]

Microscopic examination reveals uniform, typically clear, generally rounded cells arranged diffusely (Figure 2.5), in nests (Figures 2.6, 2.7), or in cords (Figure 2.8) separated by a collagenous stroma, which may be prominent (Figure 2.7). In some cases, the cytoplasm has become condensed to form a thick, eosinophilic perinuclear rim with separation of the cells from one another (Figure 2.8). Rarely, the tumor cells form irregular (Figure 2.9), as well as rounded (Figure 2.10), glandlike spaces[32] or solid-tubular structures (Figure 2.11).[33] Involvement of the rete testis in a pagetoid fashion is sometimes prominent (Figure 2.12). The stroma is almost always infiltrated by lymphocytes, which are also characteristically sprinkled among the tumor cells to varying extents (Figure 2.13). The lymphocytic infiltrate varies in prominence from case to case, with lymphoid follicles occasionally being present (Figure 2.14); plasma cells are rarely seen. An additional frequent feature of the stroma is a granulomatous reaction, with or without Langhans' giant cells (Figure 2.15). The granulomas are discrete and rounded in some cases (Figure 2.16), but a more diffuse granulomatous infiltrate is present in other cases (Figure 2.15). The granulomas may undergo central necrosis; in rare tumors, the granulomatous reaction is extensive enough to obscure the seminoma cells, leading to an erroneous diagnosis of tuberculosis or sarcoid. In one study,[34] 40% of seminomas had at least focal granulomatous infiltration, and in almost half these cases the infiltrate was marked. Granulomas are much less frequent in nonseminomatous germ cell tumors.[10]

Diffuse areas of necrosis with ghost outlines of cells may be seen in seminomas (Figure 2.17). The necrotic foci may be surrounded by palisaded histiocytes.[35] Occasional seminomas are replaced, completely or in part, by hyalinized fibrous tissue (Figure 2.18).

Seminoma cells generally have clear cytoplasm and distinct cell borders (Figure 2.13). PAS stains disclose abundant intracytoplasmic glycogen, with rare exceptions (Figure 2.19). The nuclei are typically central or slightly eccentric and are round, with focal flattening of their contours (Figure 2.20). One or a few prominent nucleoli are usually present (Figure 2.20). Mitotic figures are generally plentiful (Figure 2.20). In one study, there were three or more mitotic figures per high-power field in 87% of the cases.[17]

The seminoma is unusually vulnerable to improper fixation. The nuclei may swell (Figure 2.21), particularly in peripheral portions of the tissue sections, or they may shrink, becoming smudgy with loss of detail; occasionally they undergo extreme shrinkage, appearing as elongated, densely staining threads (Figure 2.22). In such cases, the uniformity of the tumor, its lymphocytic infiltrate, and the presence of a granulomatous reaction may provide important clues to the diagnosis.

The syncytiotrophoblast cells that are present in occasional seminomas (Figure 2.23) may contain abundant cytoplasm and relatively few nuclei or may be composed of closely packed uniform nuclei with relatively scanty cytoplasm (Figure 2.24); the cytoplasm may contain vacuoles of varying sizes. The presence of these cells should not lead to the misdiagnosis of choriocarcinoma, which contains cytotrophoblastic cells, intermediate trophoblastic cells, or both, as well as syncytiotrophoblastic cells. The latter cells are identified much more easily by immunohistochemical staining for hCG (Figure 2.25) than they are in routine sections. Typical seminomas must also be distinguished from spermatocytic seminomas (see below), embryonal carcinomas (see page 38), yolk sac tumors (see page 40), and lymphomas (see page 156).

Immunohistochemical staining may be helpful in confirming the diagnosis of seminoma in difficult cases. The tumor cells are characteristically positive for placental-like alkaline phosphatase,[36] neuron-specific enolase,[37] and vimentin[38] (Figure 2.26). They are usually negative for low–molecular weight cytokeratins,[39] but they may be positive either focally or diffusely.[40,41] The cytoplasm is negative for α-fetoprotein (AFP) and is almost always negative for hCG.[41]

The seminoma has an excellent prognosis. When it spreads as seminoma, it remains curable in almost all cases because of its generally low stage, its marked radiosensitivity, and its excellent response to combination chemotherapy. The metastases, however, are occasionally of a more highly malignant germ cell tumor type; in such cases, the prognosis depends on the nature of the latter.

Spermatocytic Seminoma

Two percent to 5% of seminomas are of the spermatocytic type.[42–45] These tumors, which have been described only in the testis, are composed mainly of cells resembling spermatogonia, with focal differentiation into larger cells that suggest primary spermatocytes in routine sections. DNA studies, however, have not revealed a haploid number of chromosomes in their nuclei, raising a question about their spermatocytic nature.[46] These tumors occur in an older age group than typical seminomas, with one half to two thirds of the patients being over 50 years of age. Bilateral involvement is seen in approximately 8% of the cases.[45] Spermatocytic seminomas also differ from typical seminomas in the appearance of their sectioned surfaces, which are typically pale yellow and edematous or gelatinous (Figure 2.27), sometimes with cyst formation; hemorrhage is an occasional finding (Figure 2.28).

Microscopic examination shows a number of features that differ from those of the typical seminoma. The tumor cells lack the striking uniformity of typical seminoma cells. Three types of cell are recognizable (Figure 2.29). The most common type approximates the typical seminoma cell in size but has denser cytoplasm that is free of glycogen and uniform, perfectly round nuclei (Figure 2.30). Scattered among these cells are smaller, degenerating cells with dense, homogenous nuclei (Figure 2.30). The largest cells, which have been likened to primary spermatocytes, occur singly or in small clusters and contain very large nuclei (Figure 2.30) with chromatin that may have a filamentous quality. Many of the nuclei, especially the larger ones, contain single prominent nucleoli, and multinucleated cells may be seen. Mitotic figures are typically numerous. The stroma is commonly edematous or myxoid, corresponding to the edematous or gelatinous appearance seen on gross examination (Figure 2.31). The testicular tubules, sometimes at a distance from the main tumor mass, are commonly occupied by spermatocytic seminoma in situ (Figure 2.32). The spermatocytic seminoma is never admixed with either typical seminoma or nonseminomatous germ cell tumors, and lacks a lymphocytic or granulomatous infiltrate in its stroma. Finally, unlike the typical seminoma, the spermatocytic type is negative for placental-like alkaline phosphatase and other antigens that can be demonstrated immunohistochemically in typical seminomas.[47]

The spermatocytic seminoma is almost always clinically benign, with only one documented case of metastasis (to para-aortic lymph nodes) in which the typical morphologic features of the tumor were present.[48] Seven cases of sarcomatous transformation have been reported;[49,50], in five of these cases the sarcomatous component was nonspecific (Figure 2.33), but in the remaining two it had the features of rhabdomyosarcoma (Figures 2.34, 2.35). Most of the tumors with sarcomatous change have metastasized as sarcomas by both lymphatic and hematogenous routes.

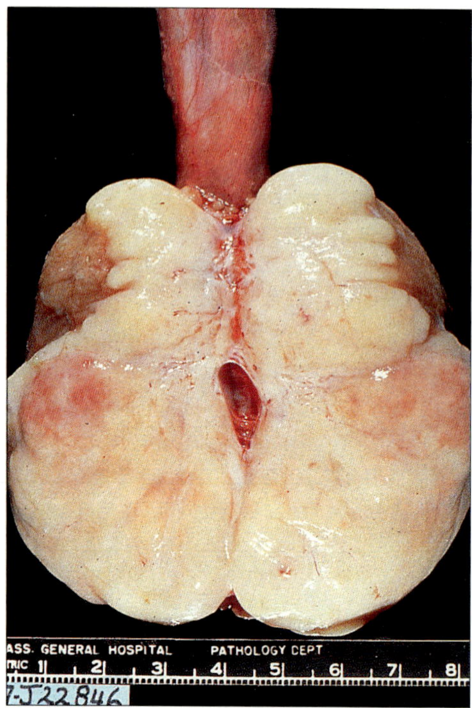

Figure 2.1 Seminoma. The neoplastic tissue is lobulated and cream colored, with focal hemorrhage, and has a soft, bulging appearance.

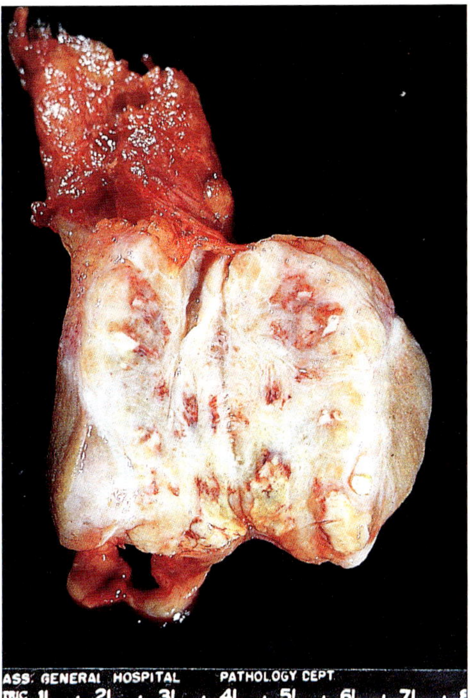

Figure 2.2 Seminoma. Necrotic and focally hemorrhagic islands of tumor are widely separated by abundant fibrous stroma.

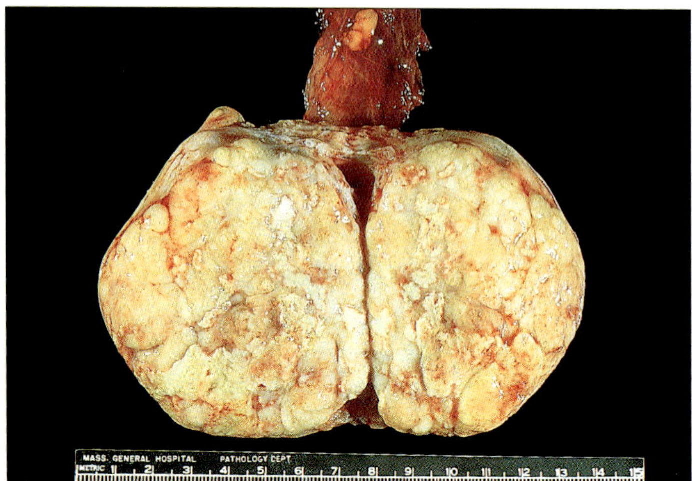

Figure 2.3 Seminoma. Extensive necrosis is present.

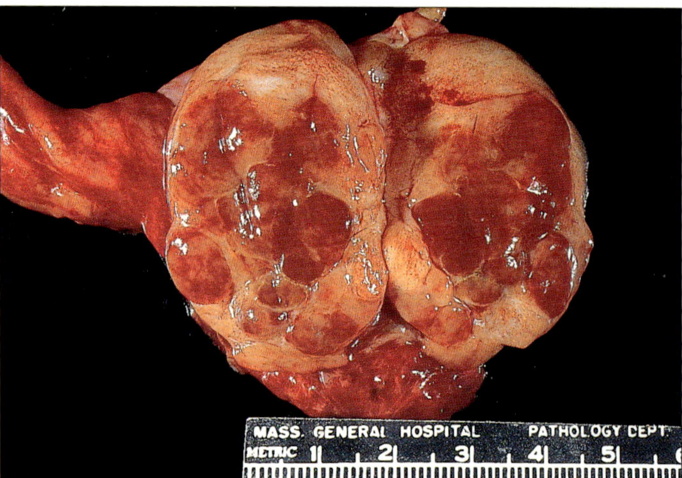

Figure 2.4 Seminoma. The tumor is lobulated, with extensive hemorrhage in most of the lobules.

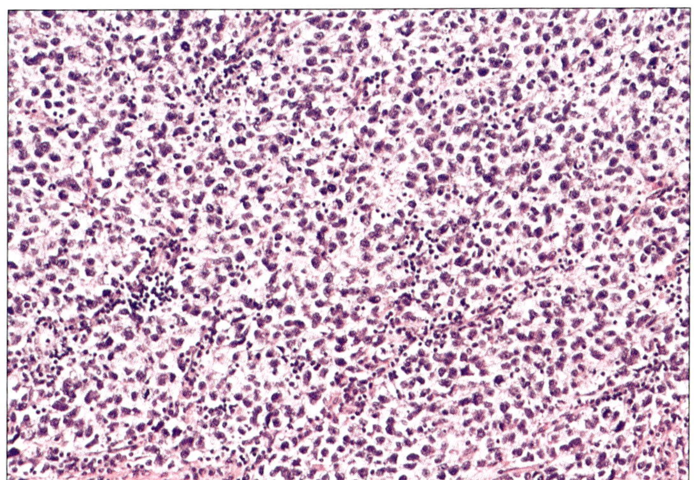

Figure 2.5 Seminoma. The tumor cells are arranged diffusely. Lymphocytic infiltration occurs mainly along vascular septa.

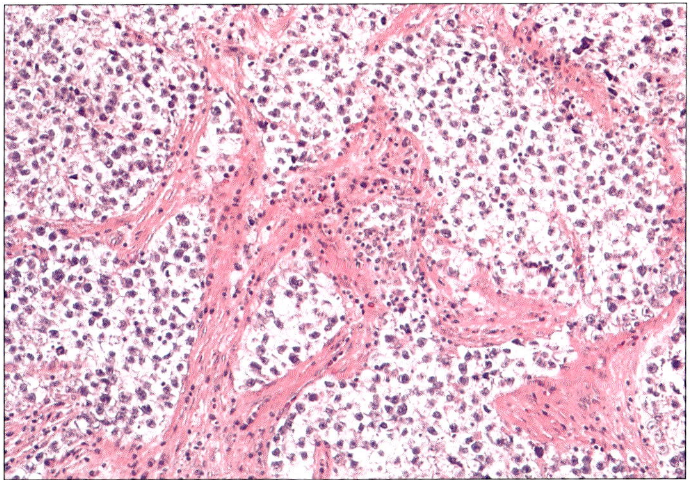

Figure 2.6 Seminoma. The neoplastic cells are arranged in irregular nests separated by fibrous septa.

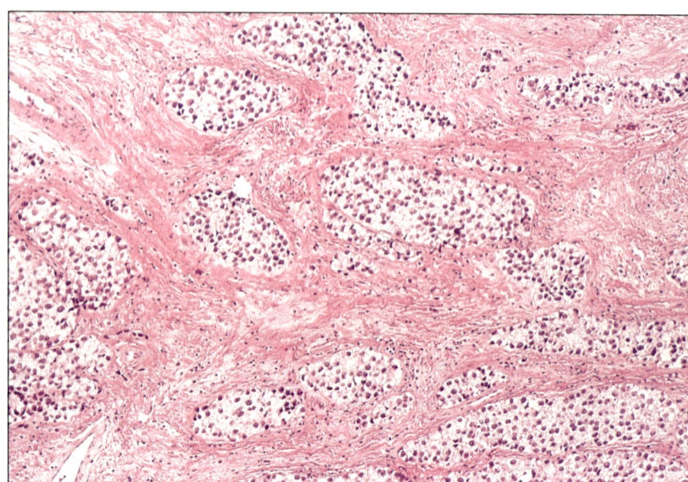

Figure 2.7 Seminoma. Nests of neoplastic cells are separated by abundant fibrous stroma.

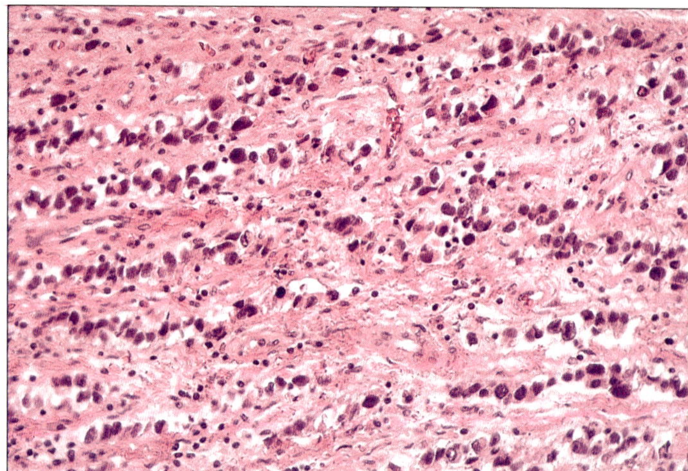

Figure 2.8 Seminoma. The neoplastic cells are arranged in thin cords separated by fibrous stroma containing scattered lymphocytes. The cytoplasm of the tumor cells has retracted around the nucleus, separating the cells from one another.

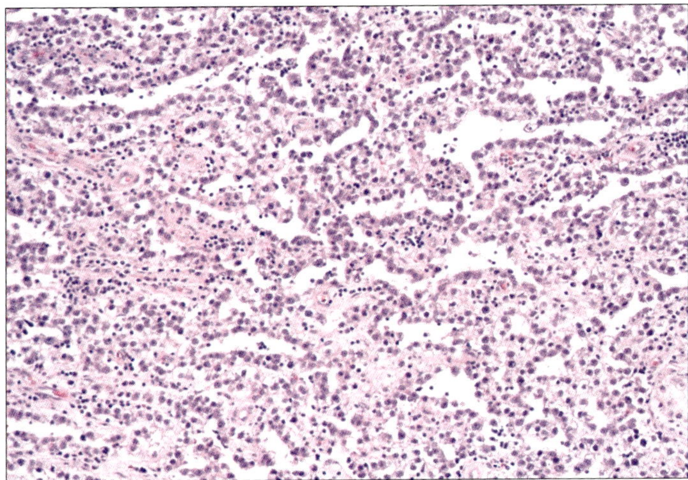

Figure 2.9 Seminoma. The neoplastic cells are arranged around irregular anastomosing spaces.

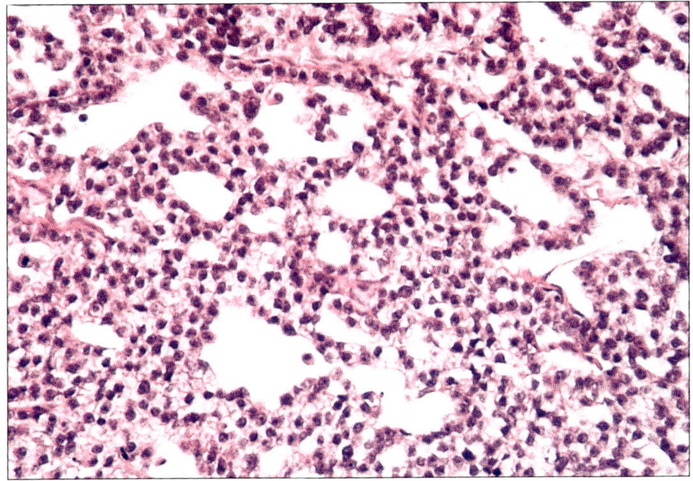

Figure 2.10 Seminoma. Several glandlike spaces are present.

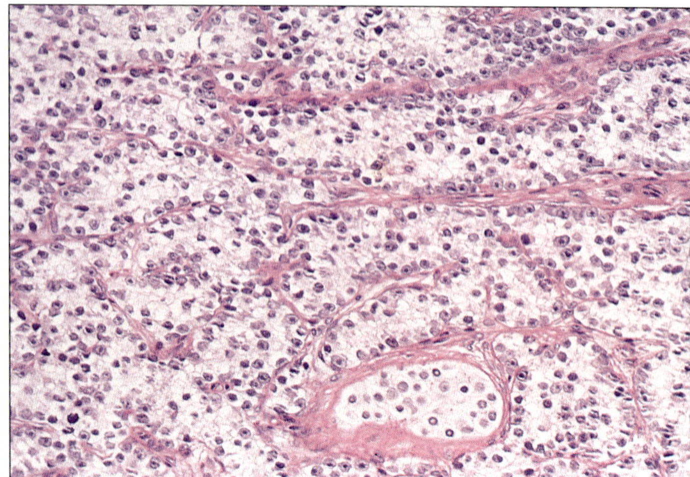

Figure 2.11 Seminoma. The tumor cells form solid tubules with most of the nuclei at the periphery.

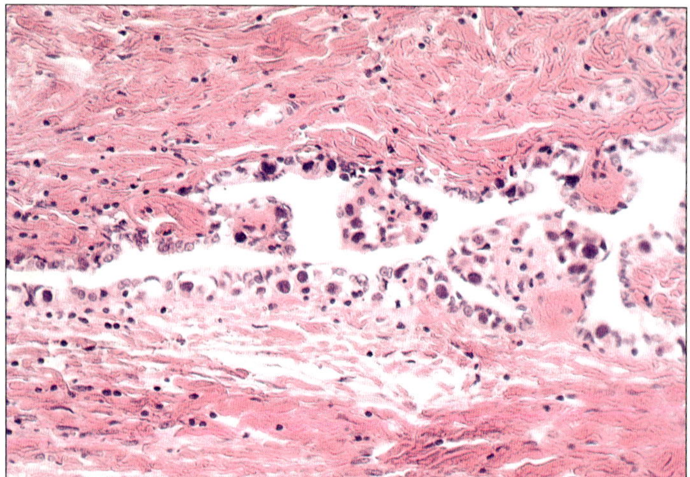

Figure 2.12 Seminoma. There is pagetoid spread along the rete testis.

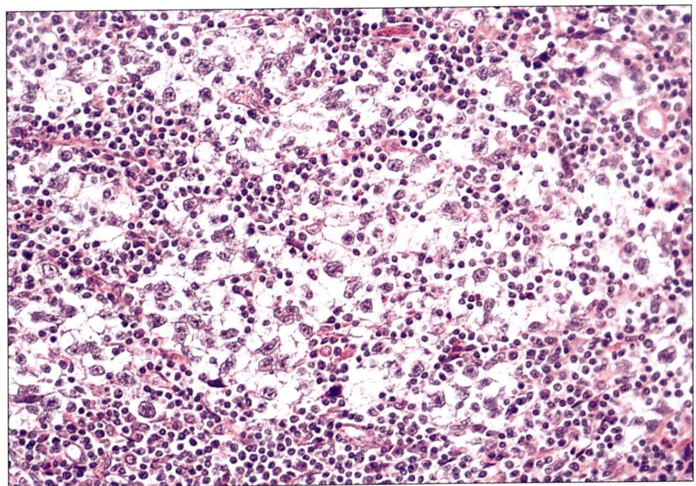

Figure 2.13 Seminoma. Numerous lymphocytes are present among the tumor cells, which are polyhedral and have abundant clear cytoplasm and distinct cell membranes.

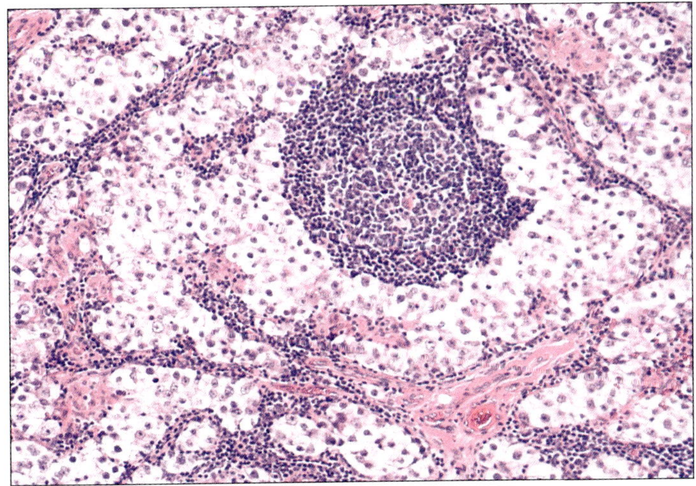

Figure 2.14 Seminoma with prominent lymphoid follicle.

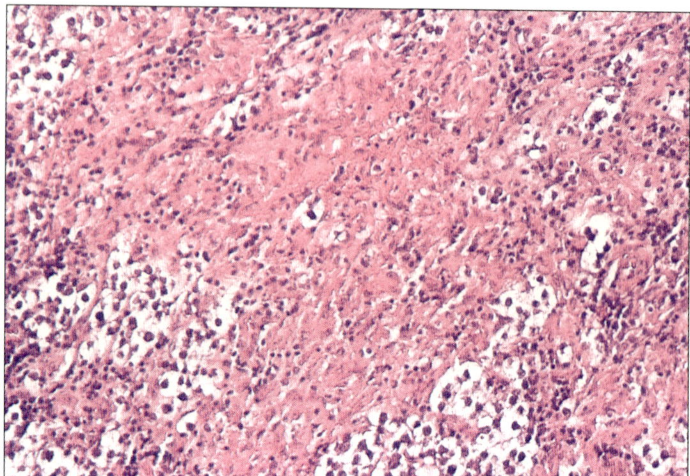

Figure 2.15 Seminoma. There is a diffuse granulomatous reaction in the stroma.

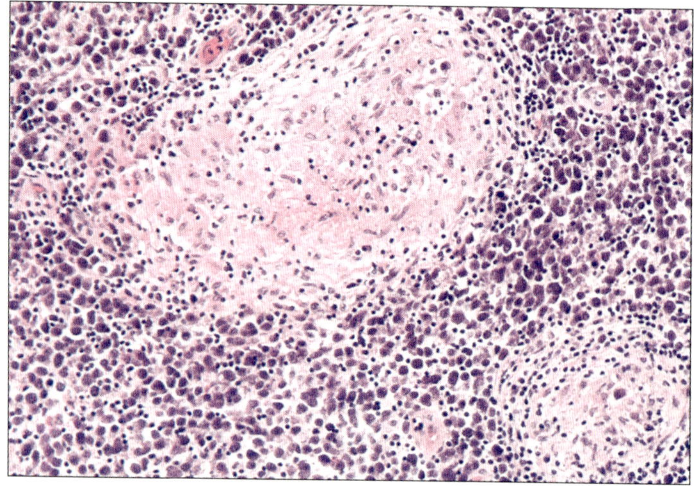

Figure 2.16 Seminoma. Two discrete granulomas are present.

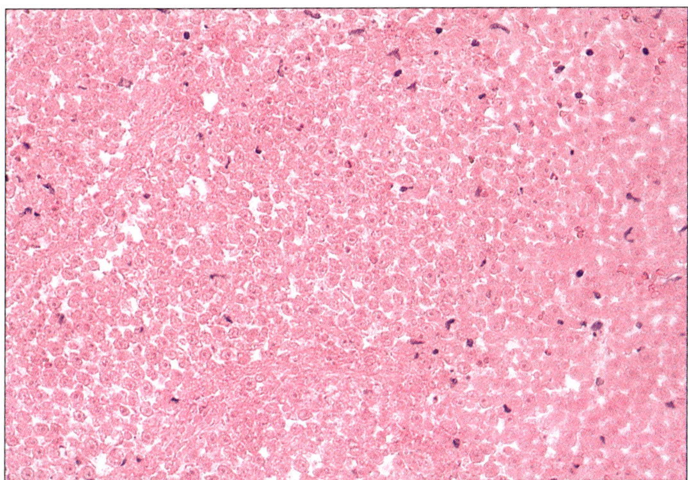

Figure 2.17 Seminoma. Ghost outlines of the neoplastic cells are visible in a diffuse area of necrosis.

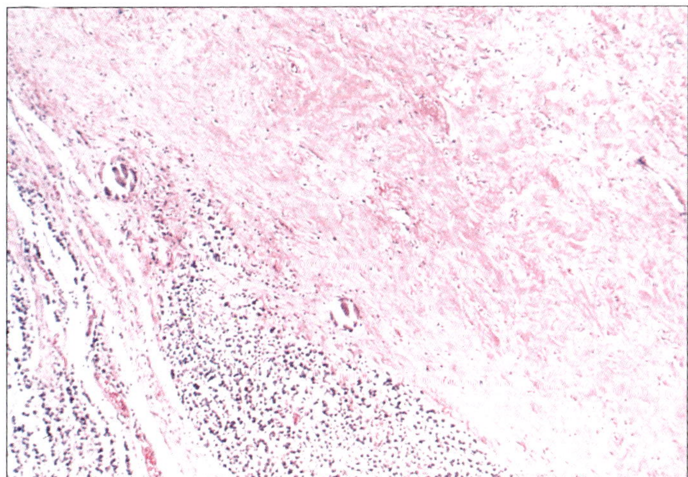

Figure 2.18 Seminoma. Massive hyalinized scar has replaced most of the tumor.

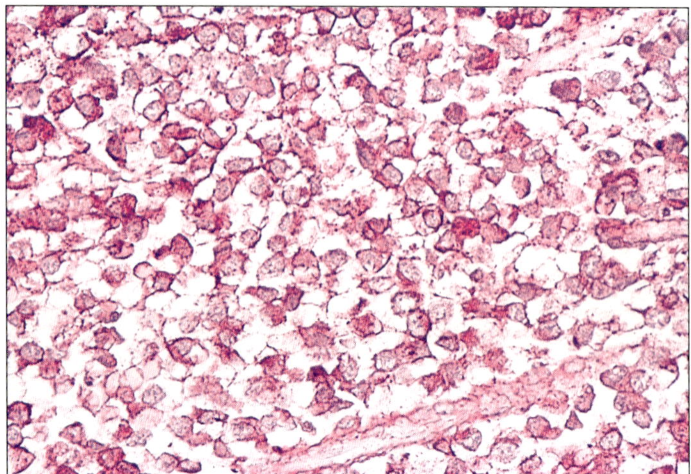

Figure 2.19 Seminoma. PAS stain shows fine intracellular glycogen granules.

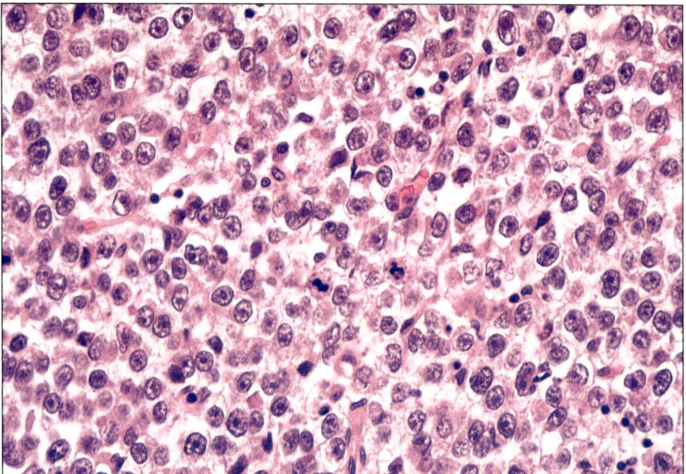

Figure 2.20 Seminoma. The neoplastic nuclei are irregularly rounded and contain prominent nucleoli; several mitotic figures are visible.

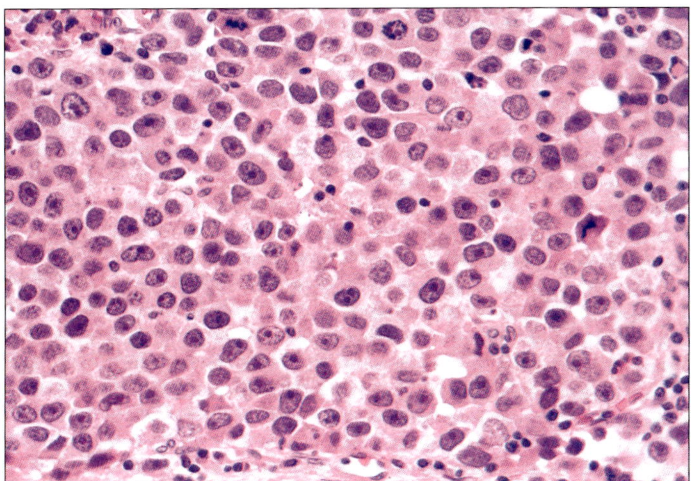

Figure 2.21 There is artifactual nuclear swelling in a section from the periphery of a seminoma. This change should not result in a misdiagnosis of embryonal carcinoma.

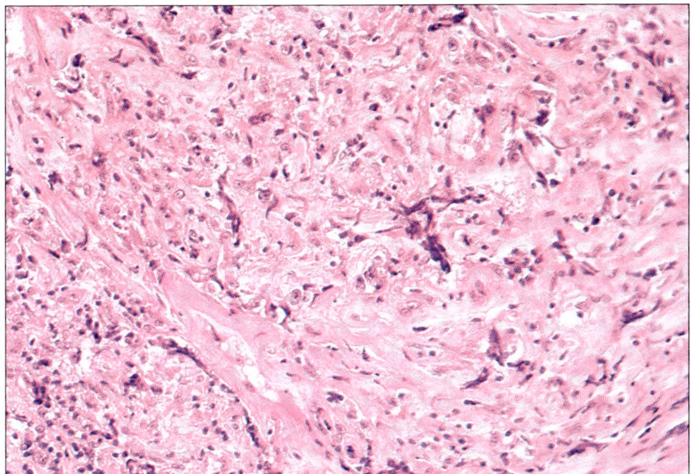

Figure 2.22 Seminoma. There is artifactual shrinkage of the neoplastic cells into threadlike forms separated by abundant fibrous stroma.

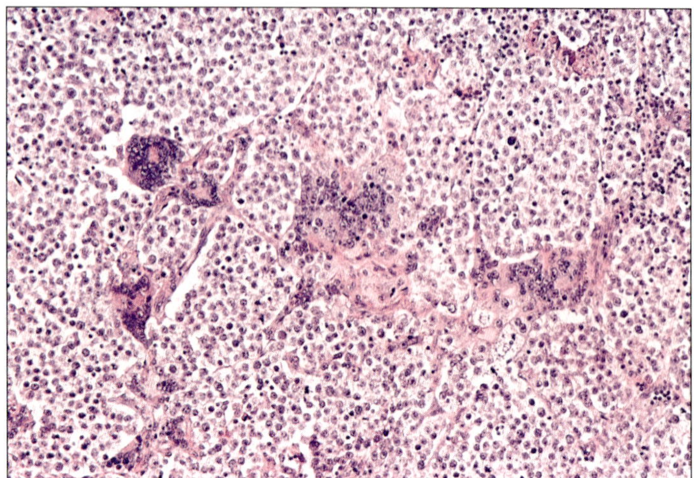

Figure 2.23 Seminoma. Syncytiotrophoblast cells containing large numbers of nuclei are present.

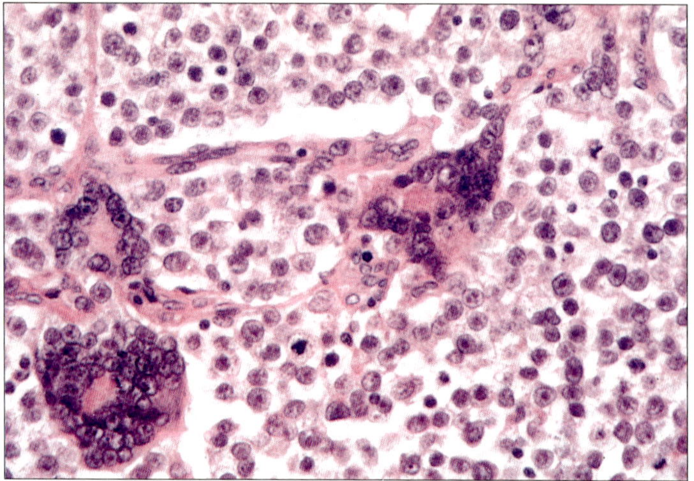

Figure 2.24 Seminoma with syncytiotrophoblast cells.

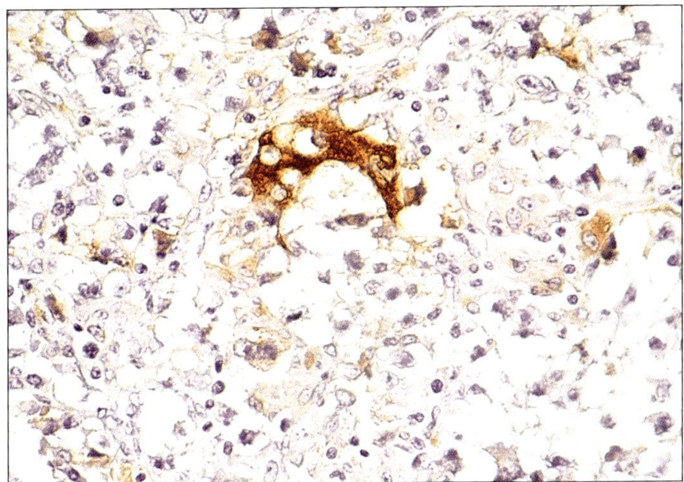

Figure 2.25 Seminoma with syncytiotrophoblast cells. The cytoplasm of a large syncytiotrophoblast cell is stained immunohistochemically for chorionic gonadotropin.

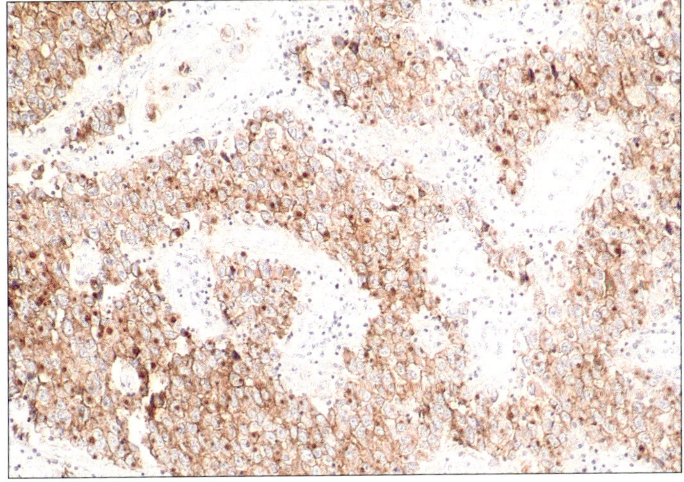

Figure 2.26 Seminoma. The tumor cells are stained immunohistochemically for vimentin.

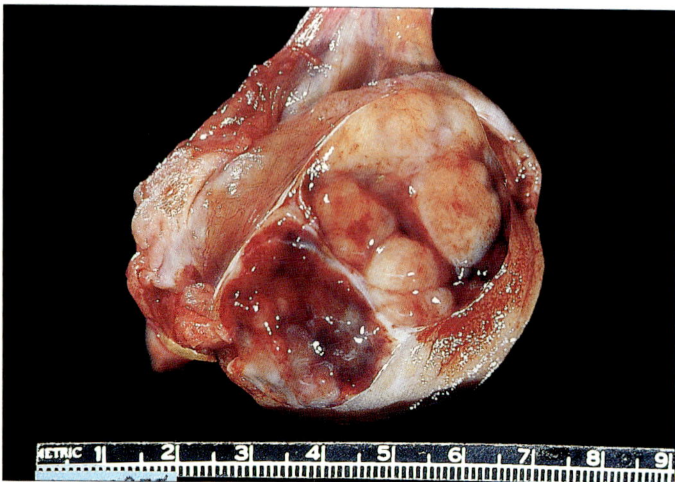

Figure 2.27 Spermatocytic seminoma. The neoplastic tissue has a gelatinous, focally hemorrhagic appearance.

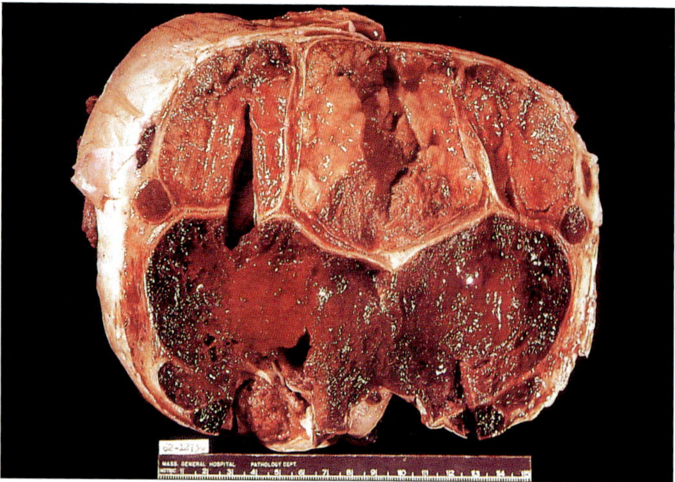

Figure 2.28 Spermatocytic seminoma. The neoplastic tissue is lobulated by fibrous septa and is extensively hemorrhagic in the lower portion of its sectioned surface.

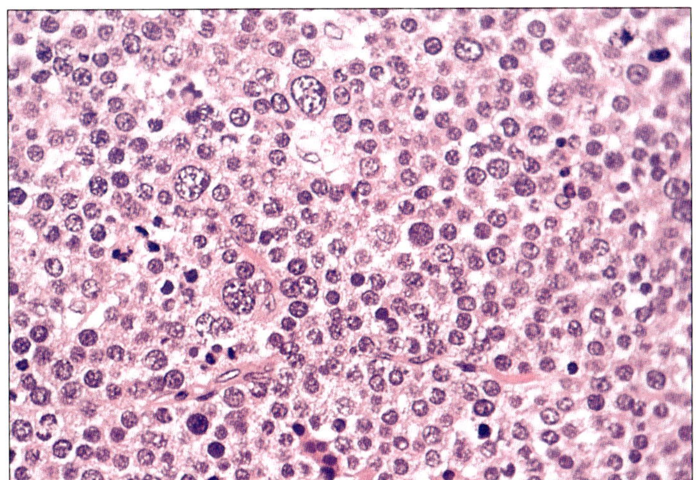

Figure 2.29 Spermatocytic seminoma. The nuclei vary markedly in size, are perfectly rounded, and contain abundant cytoplasm. There is no lymphocytic infiltration.

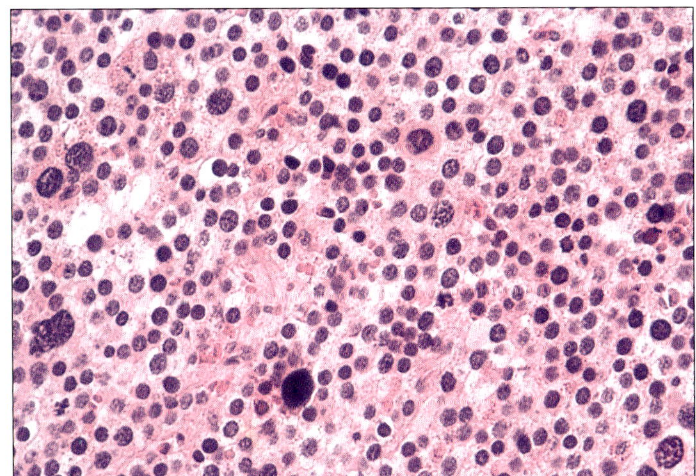

Figure 2.30 Spermatocytic seminoma. Three types of nuclei are visible: a few large, rounded forms; predominant medium-sized, round nuclei; and round, uniformly dark, shrunken nuclei.

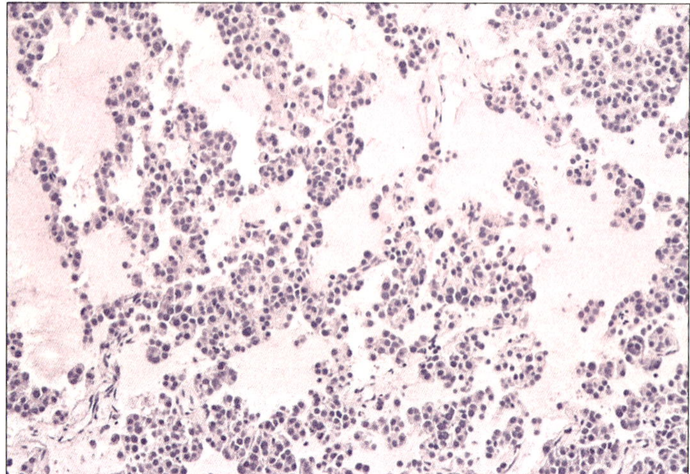

Figure 2.31 Spermatocytic seminoma. The stroma is myxoid, corresponding to the characteristic gelatinous appearance of the tumor on gross examination.

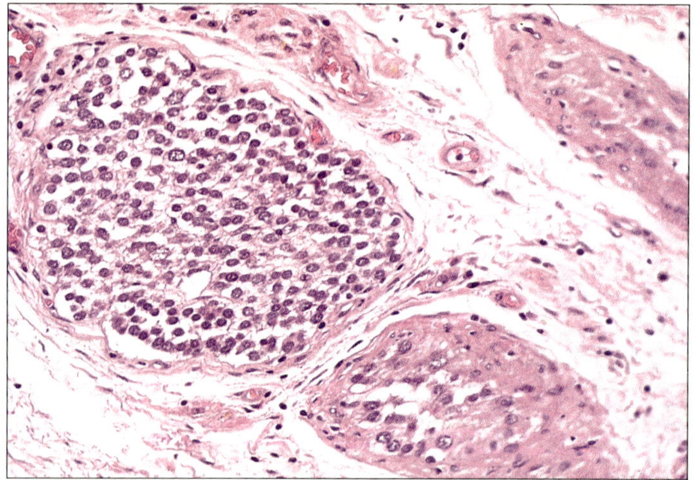

Figure 2.32 Spermatocytic seminoma, intratubular. This tubule was at a distance from the main tumor mass.

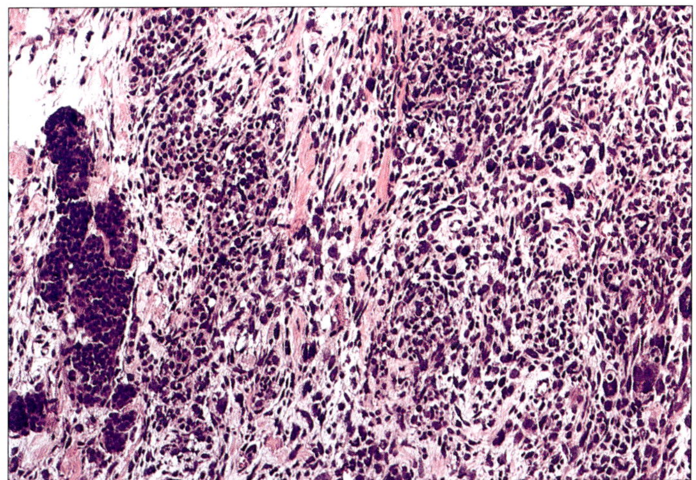

Figure 2.33 Spermatocytic seminoma with sarcoma. Typical spermatocytic seminoma is seen at the left edge of the picture. Most of the tumor is composed of sarcoma.

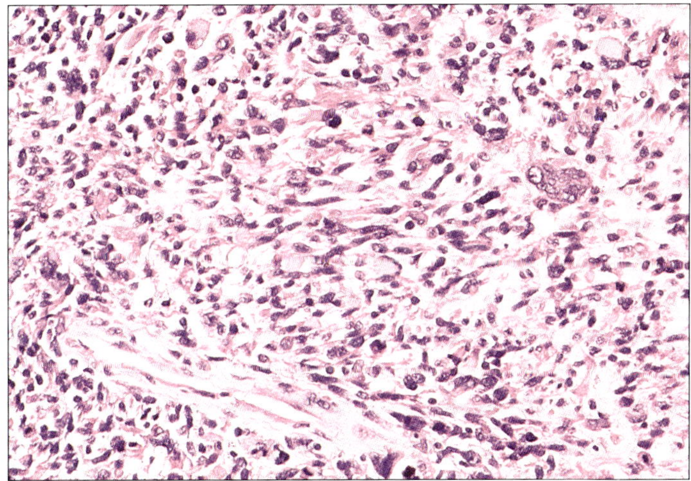

Figure 2.34 Spermatocytic seminoma with rhabdomyosarcoma.

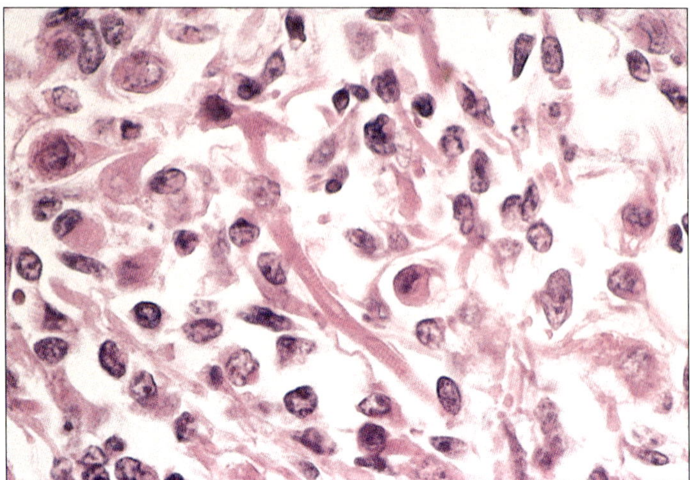

Figure 2.35 Spermatocytic seminoma with rhabdomyosarcoma. A strap cell with cross-striations is seen in the rhabdomyosarcomatous component of the tumor.

References

1. Mostofi FK, Price EB Jr. *Atlas of Tumor Pathology*, Second Series, Fascicle 8. *Tumors of the Male Genital System.* Washington, DC, Armed Forces Institute of Pathology, 1973.
2. Pugh RCB. *Pathology of the Testis.* Boston, Blackwell Scientific Publications Inc, 1976.
3. Von Hochstetter AR, Hedinger CE. The differential diagnosis of testicular germ cell tumors in theory and practice: A critical analysis of two major systems of classification and review of 389 cases. *Virchows Arch A* 396:247–277, 1982.
4. Silverberg E, Lubera JA. Cancer statistics. *CA* 38:5–22, 1988.
5. Silverberg E. Cancer in young adults (ages 15 to 34). *CA* 32:32–42, 1982.
6. Dixon FJ, Moore RA. Testicular tumors: A clinicopathological study. *Cancer* 6:427–454, 1953.
7. Morrison AS. Cryptorchidism, hernia, and cancer of the testis. *JNCI* 56:731–733, 1976.
8. Giwercman A, Grindsted J, Hansen B, Jensen OM, Skakkebaek NE. Testicular cancer risk in boys with maldescended testis: A cohort study. *J Urol* 138:1214–1216, 1987.
9. Teppo L. Epidemiology of testicular neoplasms. In: *Pathology of the Testis and its Adnexa,* Talerman A, Roth LM, eds. *Contemporary Issues in Surgical Pathology,* vol 7. New York, Churchill Livingstone, 1986, chap 1.
10. Jacobsen GK, Barlebo H, Olsen J, et al. Testicular germ cell tumours in Denmark 1976–1980: Pathology of 1058 consecutive cases. *Acta Radiol Oncol* 23:239–247, 1984.
11. Scully RE, Parham AR. Testicular tumors: I. Seminoma and teratoma. *Arch Pathol Lab Med* 45:581–607, 1948.
12. Babaian RJ, Zagars GK. Testicular seminoma: The M. D. Anderson experience, an analysis of pathological and patient characteristics and treatment recommendations. *J Urol* 139:311–315, 1988.
13. Parkinson C, Beilby JOW. Features of prognostic significance in testicular germ cell tumors. *J Clin Pathol* 30:113–119, 1977.
14. Schultz HP, Von Der Maase H, Rorth M, et al. Testicular seminoma in Denmark 1976–1980. *Acta Radiol Oncol* 23:263–270, 1984.
15. Percarpio B, Clements JC, McLeod DG, Sorgen SD, Cardinale FS. Anaplastic seminoma: An analysis of 77 patients. *Cancer* 43:2510–2513, 1979.
16. Cockburn AG, Vugrin D, Batata M, Hajdu S, Whitmore WF. Poorly differentiated (anaplastic) seminoma of the testis. *Cancer* 53:1991–1994, 1984.
17. Von Hochstetter AR. Mitotic count in seminomas: An unreliable criterion for distinguishing between classical and anaplastic types. *Virchows Arch A* 390:63–69, 1981.
18. Zuckman MH, Williams G, Levin HS. Mitosis counting in seminoma: An exercise of questionable significance. *Hum Pathol* 19:329–335, 1988.

19. Hedinger C, von Hochstetter AR, Egloff B. Seminoma with syncytiotrophoblastic giant cells: A special form of seminoma. *Virchows Arch A* 383:59–67, 1979.

20. Von Hochstetter AR, Sigg C, Saremaslani P, Hedinger C. The significance of giant cells in human testicular seminomas. *Virchows Arch A* 407:309–322, 1985.

21. Butcher DN, Gregory WM, Gunter PA, Masters JRW, Parkinson MD. The biological and clinical significance of HCG containing cells in seminoma. *Br J Cancer* 51:473–478, 1985.

22. Weissbach L, Altwein JE, Stiens R. Germinal testicular tumors in childhood: A report of observations and literature review. *Eur Urol* 10:73–85, 1984.

23. Ferguson JD. Tumours of the testis. *Br J Urol* 34:407–421, 1962.

24. Scully RE. Testicular tumors with endocrine manifestations. In: *Endocrinology*, de Groot LJ, Besser GM, Cahill GF, et al, (eds). Philadelphia, WB Saunders Co, 1989, vol 3, chap 134.

25. Mann AS. Bilateral exophthalmos in seminoma. *J Clin Endocrinol Metab* 27:1500–1502, 1967.

26. Taylor JB, Solomon DH, Levine RE, Ehrlich RM. Exophthalmos in seminoma: Regression with steroids and orchiectomy. *JAMA* 240:860–861, 1978.

27. Miles, BJ, Kiesling VJ Jr, Belville WD. Bilateral synchronous germ cell tumors. *J Urol* 133:679–680, 1985.

28. Kristianslund S, Fossa S, Kjellevold K. Bilateral malignant testicular germ cell cancer. *Br J Urol* 58:60–63, 1986.

29. Scheiber K, Ackermann D, Studer UE. Bilateral testicular germ cell tumors: A report of 20 cases. *J Urol* 138:73–76, 1987.

30. Thompson J, Williams CJ, Whitehouse JMA, Mead GM. Bilateral testicular germ cell tumours: An increasing incidence and prevention by chemotherapy. *Br J Urol* 62:374–376, 1988.

31. Jacobsen GK, Talerman A. *Atlas of Germ Cell Tumors.* Copenhagen, Munksgaard, 1989.

32. Damjanov I, Niejadlik DC, Rabuffo, JV, Donadio JA. Cribriform and sclerosing seminoma devoid of lymphoid infiltrates. *Arch Pathol Lab* Med 104:527–530, 1980.

33. Young RH, Finlayson N, Scully RE. Tubular seminoma: Report of a case. *Arch Pathol Lab Med* 113:414–416, 1989.

34. Thackray AC. Seminoma: The pathology of testicular tumors. *Br J Urol* 36(suppl):12–27, 1964.

35. Friedman NB, Moore RA. Tumors of the testis: A report of 922 cases. *Mil Surg* 99:573–593, 1946.

36. Manivel JC, Jessurun J, Wick MR, Dehner LP. Placental alkaline phosphatase immunoreactivity in testicular germ-cell neoplasms. *Am J Surg Pathol* 11:21–29, 1987.

37. Kuzmits R, Schernthaner G, Krisch K. Serum neuron-specific enolase: A marker for response to therapy in seminoma. *Cancer* 60:1017–1021, 1987.

38. Padfield CJH, MacLennan KA. Immunostaining for cytokeratin and vimentin in seminoma and embryonal carcinoma. *J Pathol* 156:197a, 1988.

39. Battifora H, Sheibani K, Tubbs RR, Kopinski MI, Sun T-T. Antikeratin antibodies in tumor diagnosis: Distinction between seminoma and embryonal carcinoma. *Cancer* 54:843–848, 1984.

40. Eglen DE, Ulbright TM. The differential diagnosis of yolk sac tumor and seminoma: Usefulness of cytokeratin, alpha-fetoprotein, and alpha-l-antitrypsin immunoperoxidase reactions. *Am J Clin Pathol* 88:328–332, 1987.

41. Jacobsen GK, Jacobsen M. Alpha-fetoprotein (AFP) and human chorionic gonadotropin in testicular germ cell tumours: A prospective immunohistochemical study. *Acta Path Microbiol Immunol Scand A* 91:165–176, 1983.

42. Scully RE. Spermatocytic seminoma of the testis: A report of 3 cases and review of the literature. *Cancer* 14:788–794, 1961.

43. Rosai J, Silber I, Khodadoust K. Spermatocytic seminoma: I. Clinicopathologic study of six cases and review of the literature. *Cancer* 24:92–102, 1969.

44. Walter P. Séminome spermatocytaire: Etude de 8 observations et revue de la littérature. *Virchows Arch A* 386:175–187, 1980.

45. Talerman A. Spermatocytic seminoma: Clinicopathological study of 22 cases. *Cancer* 45:2169–2176, 1980.

46. Talerman A, Fu YS, Okagaki T. Spermatocytic seminoma: Ultrastructural and microspectrophotometric observations. *Lab Invest* 51:343–349, 1984.

47. Aguirre P, Scully RE, Dayal Y, DeLellis R. Placental-like alkaline phosphatase in germ cell tumors of the ovary and testis. *Lab Invest* 52:2A, 1985.

48. Matoska J, Ondrus D, Hornak M. Metastatic spermatocytic seminoma: A case report with light microscopic, ultrastructural, and immunohistochemical findings. *Cancer* 62:1197–1201, 1988.

49. True LD, Otis CN, Delprado W, Scully RE, Rosai J. Spermatocytic seminoma of testis with sarcomatous transformation: A report of five cases. *Am J Surg Pathol* 12:75–82, 1988.

50. Floyd C, Ayala AG, Logothetis CJ, Silva EG. Spermatocytic seminoma with associated sarcoma of the testis. *Cancer* 61:409–414, 1988.

Germ Cell Tumors: Nonseminomatous Tumors, Occult Tumors, Effects of Chemotherapy

3

Embryonal Carcinoma

Embryonal carcinoma is the second most frequent form of pure testicular germ cell tumor, accounting for approximately 20% of the cases.[1] This tumor has a younger peak age incidence than seminoma, being most common between 25 and 35 years of age. It is exceptionally rare before puberty and in men over 50 years of age. The patients usually present with testicular swelling, sometimes accompanied by pain, but occasionally gynecomastia is the initial complaint, and some patients present with symptoms related to metastatic spread. An undescended testis or a history of cryptorchidism is less often present than in cases of seminoma. The tumors are unilateral with rare exceptions. On gross examination, they are typically smaller and have a more variegated appearance than the seminoma;[2] sectioning discloses white to yellow, solid, often granular-appearing tissue (Figure 3.1); areas of necrosis and hemorrhage are common. Extensive fibrosis is occasionally seen (Figure 3.2).

Microscopic examination reveals primitive epithelial cells that may grow in solid (Figure 3.3), glandular (Figure 3.4), tubular, or papillary patterns (Figure 3.5); areas of necrosis are more common and generally more extensive than in the seminoma.[3–6] The cytoplasm of the tumor cells varies from amphophilic (Figure 3.3) to slightly basophilic to clear, and is generally abundant and finely granular; the large, hyperchromatic, pleomorphic nuclei typically contain one or more prominent eosinophilic nucleoli (Figure 3.3) and exhibit considerable mitotic activity (Figure 3.6); occasionally the nuclei are very large and clear (Figure 3.6). Although the cells are usually much larger, darker, and less uniform than those of a seminoma, they resemble closely seminoma cells in some cases. Syncytiotrophoblast cells are often scattered among the embryonal carcinoma cells (Figure 3.7). The stroma is usually relatively inconspicuous, but rarely it is prominent; it has a nonspecific fibrous character in most cases, but may be cellular and immature (Figure 3.8); the presence of cellular mesenchyme is considered compatible with the diagnosis of embryonal carcinoma and does not warrant a designation of teratoma.

Embryonal carcinomas must be distinguished from seminomas, yolk sac tumors (see page 40), and lymphomas (see page 152). Differentiation from seminomas is rarely a problem because of the almost invariable absence of gland formation and papillae in seminomas, the uniformity of seminoma cells and their nuclei (which are smaller and less atypical than those of embryonal carcinomas), and the characteristic lymphocytic infiltrate and granulomas of the seminoma. It should be mentioned, however, that the latter are also seen rarely in embryonal carcinomas. Difficulty in differential diagnosis may arise when, exceptionally, the seminoma forms glandlike spaces or its nuclei are artifactually enlarged, or when the embryonal carcinoma has a solid component of relatively small, clear cells that lack the usual high degree of nuclear atypicality. Almost always, a combination of architectural and cytologic features enables one to make the correct diagnosis. Immunohistochemical staining may help to confirm the diagnosis of embryonal carcinoma. Like the seminoma, the embryonal carcinoma is positive for placental-like alkaline phosphatase and neuron-specific enolase, but unlike the usual seminoma, it stains regularly for low–molecular weight cytokeratins (Figure 3.9).[7,8] Scattered syncytiotrophoblast cells are present more frequently than in the seminoma, and in addition, isolated cells indistinguishable on routine staining from their neighbors may be stained for hCG or AFP.

The embryonal carcinoma is more highly malignant than the seminoma, presenting at a more advanced stage in a high proportion of the cases and much more frequently spreading via the bloodstream (Figure 3.10). It almost always metastasizes as embryonal carcinoma or choriocarcinoma.[2] The embryonal carcinoma is considerably less radiosensitive than the seminoma, but can be cured by surgical removal with or without combination chemotherapy in almost 90% of cases.[6]

Yolk Sac Tumor (Endodermal Sinus Tumor)

The yolk sac tumor may be seen in the testis in pure form,[9–18] or as a component of a mixed germ cell tumor.[19–21] The pure tumor, which is encountered in infancy and childhood in the great majority of cases, accounts for approximately two thirds of all testicular tumors in that age group,[18,22] but for less than 2% of all germ cell tumors. Eighty percent of such tumors occur in the first two years of life,[13] with a progressively decreasing incidence with increasing age.

Gross examination typically reveals a mass 2 to 4 cm in diameter that has generally replaced most of the parenchyma. Sectioning discloses predominantly solid, soft, white, gray or pale yellow tissue (Figure 3.11); cystic degeneration as well as foci of necrosis and hemorrhage may be present.

The most frequently encountered histologic pattern, present at least focally in most of the tumors, is reticular (Figure 3.12) or microcystic (Figure 3.13), characterized by a loose meshwork of irregular spaces lined by flat, cuboidal, or columnar cells of primitive appearance. In many cases, solitary papillae with a connective tissue core containing a central vessel project into some of the spaces (Figure 3.14); the papillae may be round or elongated (Figure 3.12). These structures, known as Schiller-Duval bodies, are highly characteristic of yolk sac tumor, but are often sparse or absent. Their presence was responsible for the original designation "endodermal sinus tumor" because similar papillary structures in the normal rat placenta are referred to as "endodermal sinuses." In view of their frequent absence from human tumors of yolk sac type, however, the term yolk sac tumor is now preferred as a generic designation for these neoplasms.

Other patterns of yolk sac tumors include solid (Figure 3.15), vacuolated (Figure 3.16), glandular and papillary (Figure 3.17), festoon (Figure 3.18), macrocystic, polyvesicular (Figure 3.19), and parietal (Figure 3.20). The cells in the solid areas occasionally have abundant clear cytoplasm (Figure 3.15). In the vacuolated pattern, rounded vacuoles of various sizes are present, sometimes mimicking a liposarcoma (Figure 3.16). The cysts that are present in many yolk sac tumors may vary considerably in size and are frequently lined by flattened, attenuated cells that appear deceptively benign. In areas with a polyvesicular pattern, vesicles resembling the yolk sac vesicle of the embryo are separated by mesenchyme (Figure 3.19). Some of the vesicles may show an eccentric constriction (Figure 3.19), simulating the formation of the secondary yolk sac from the primary yolk sac in the normal embryo. The epithelium lining the secondary component of the vesicle is often columnar, in contrast to the attenuated epithelium lining the primary component. Consistent with differentiation into secondary yolk sac, which develops into the gastrointestinal tract and its derivatives in the normal embryo, is the occasional presence of mucinous glands (Figure 3.21) and clusters of cells resembling hepatocytes in yolk sac tumors (Figure 3.22). Hepatoid differentiation was observed in approximately one fifth of yolk sac tumors in one series of cases.[22] The most commonly encountered cells of yolk sac tumors are of moderate to large size; they contain clear to amphophilic to slightly basophilic cytoplasm and large atypical nuclei showing slight to marked mitotic activity (Figure 3.23); these cells may resemble those of either the embryonal carcinoma or the seminoma. Occasionally, clusters of cells with scanty cytoplasm and closely packed hyperchromatic nuclei are observed (Figure 3.24). Similar cells may line glands. Rarely, the solid areas of yolk sac tumors in which the cells have abundant clear cytoplasm may simulate renal cell carcinoma (Figure 3.25). A characteristic but nonspecific feature of many yolk sac tumors is the presence of round, eosinophilic, PAS-positive, diastase-resistant hyaline globules (Figure 3.24). The stroma of yolk sac tumors may be fibrous, edematous, or myxoid (Figure 3.26), or may be composed of cellular mesenchyme. The tumor cells in yolk sac tumors almost always can be stained, at least focally, for AFP (Figure 3.27). They also can be stained for low molecular weight cytokeratin and placental-like alkaline phosphatase.[23]

Pure yolk sac tumors are usually not difficult to distinguish from other forms of germ cell tumor because of their almost exclusive occurrence in infants and young children, in whom other types of germ cell neoplasia, except for teratoma, are extremely rare. A tumor that may cause a significant problem in infancy, particularly in the neonatal period, is the juvenile granulosa cell tumor (see page 107), which may have a vacuolated pattern and in some cases contains cells with atypical nuclei. That tumor, however, typically forms follicles, lacks other patterns of yolk sac tumor, and does not stain immunohistochemically for AFP. In contrast to the juvenile granulosa cell tumor and most other germ cell tumors, yolk sac tumors are positive at least focally for AFP in the great majority of cases; the hyaline globules are usually not stained for this antigen.

The pure yolk sac tumor spreads distantly less often than the embryonal carcinoma; like the latter, it is often curable by surgical removal with or without combination chemotherapy. In one large study, 13% of the patients died of the tumor or as a result of the treatment.[18] In that series, approximately two thirds of the patients with metastatic disease were salvaged by chemotherapy, radiotherapy, or surgical removal.

Choriocarcinoma

Choriocarcinoma occurs very rarely as a pure neoplasm,[24–26] and much more often as a component of a mixed germ cell tumor. Gynecomastia or manifestations of metastatic disease may be the presenting symptom.[27] On gross examination, the pure tumor is typically hemorrhagic and smaller than other germ cell tumors (Figure 3.28). Microscopic examination shows an admixture of cytotrophoblast or intermediate trophoblast and syncytiotrophoblast characteristic of choriocarcinomas occurring elsewhere (Figure 3.29). Occasionally, the tumors are less differentiated and lack a clear biphasic pattern (Figure 3.30). The adjacent testis may show Leydig cell hyperplasia (Figure 3.31) secondary to elevated levels of hCG. The choriocarcinoma stains immunohistochemically for hCG, placental lactogen (hPL) and various placental proteins.[28] The hCG and hPL are confined to syncytiotrophoblast cells and occasional mononucleate cells that are probably intermediate trophoblast cells.[28] We have seen one trophoblastic tumor of the testis that was made up exclusively of intermediate trophoblast cells with microscopic and immunohistochemical features similar to those of the placental site trophoblastic tumor (Figures 3.32, 3.33).

In addition to being distinguished from the seminoma and embryonal carcinoma with scattered syncytiotrophoblast cells, the true choriocarcinoma should not be confused with the choriocarcinomalike tumor that may appear at metastatic sites after chemotherapy, since the latter usually stains for hCG but, unlike the choriocarcinoma, generally stains for mucin as well; it does not appear to be associated with the high levels of hCG or the sinister prognosis of true choriocarcinoma.[29]

Polyembryoma

Although structures closely resembling normal embryos, termed "embryoid bodies,"[30] are often seen in embryonal carcinomas and mixed germ cell tumors, exceedingly rare neoplasms composed entirely or predominantly of these structures are designated *polyembryoma*. Embryoid bodies in their fully developed forms are composed of an amniotic cavity, germ disc, yolk sac, extraembryonic mesenchyme, and trophoblast (Figures 3.34 to 3.36). Some of the embryoid bodies differentiate focally into mucinous tubules, clusters of cells resembling hepatocytes, neuroectodermal tubules, squamous epithelium, and mesenchymal derivatives in varying proportions.

Teratoma

Teratoma is a frequent component of a mixed germ cell tumor, but pure teratomas account for only 7% of germ cell neoplasms.[31,32] These tumors are rare after the first three decades of life, being most common in early childhood and early adult life. Even in the last two age periods, teratomas are uncommon; only eight examples were seen over a 54-year period in a large children's hospital.[33]

Teratomas are divided into mature and immature forms, with the former being composed exclusively of mature elements and the latter containing at least some immature components. The most common ovarian germ cell tumor, the dermoid cyst, is extremely rare in the testis. On gross examination, teratomas are typically relatively large. Sectioning reveals a variegated appearance with cystic and solid components in varying proportions (Figure 3.37). The cysts may be lined by white membranes resembling skin and the contents of the cysts may be keratinous (Figure 3.38), sebaceous, serous, or mucinous. The solid tissue between the cysts may contain discernible foci of cartilage, bone, and soft, tan-white tissue resembling brain tissue; occasionally black foci of retinal tissue are visible. Microscopic examination shows an admixture of ectodermal, endodermal and mesodermal elements, which may be mature (Figures 3.39, 3.40), immature (Figures 3.41, 3.42), or both. The immunohistochemical features of teratomas obviously vary widely. It is important to emphasize that endodermal tissue within these tumors often stains for AFP.

One component of a teratoma may undergo malignant transformation to form a cancer of somatic type, such as a mucinous or squamous cell carcinoma or a sarcoma (Figure 3.43),[34] but such a development is much rarer in testicular than in ovarian teratomas. These types of cancer have been reported in testicular tumors both as spontaneous events and after chemotherapy. All pure teratomas in prepubertal boys, whether mature or immature, follow a benign course. In contrast, teratomas occurring in postpubertal males, even though mature, may metastasize, occasionally as such, but sometimes in the form of a more highly malignant, nonseminomatous germ cell tumor. Perhaps because of their rarity, no correlation of the degree of differentiation of teratomas and their metastatic potential has been reported. Teratomas occurring after puberty are managed as malignant germ cell tumors, with radical orchidectomy and additional operations with or without combination chemotherapy, depending upon the presence or absence of more highly malignant tumor types in the metastases.

Carcinoid Tumor

Among the 30 reported cases of testicular carcinoid tumor, all but a few have been interpreted as being primary tumors of germ cell origin.[35]

Such an origin has been proven by finding other teratomatous elements, however, in only approximately 15% of the reported cases; therefore, it is possible that some pure carcinoid tumors judged to have been primary were actually metastatic from an occult primary tumor. The finding of intratubular germ cell neoplasia (see Chapter 4) adjacent to a carcinoid indicates that the tumor is primary in the testis. Most primary carcinoid tumors have occurred in patients in the fourth to sixth decades.[35–37] None has been reported in children, but we have seen one that occurred in a 12-year-old boy. All of the tumors have been unilateral. Symptoms of the carcinoid syndrome have been reported in only a single case.[36] Gross examination typically shows a solid, tan to white to pale yellow mass devoid of hemorrhage or necrosis. Microscopic examination discloses various combinations of insular (Figure 3.44), acinar, and trabecular patterns characteristic of this neoplasm and the cells have finely granular, acidophilic cytoplasm and round nuclei with clumped chromatin (Figure 3.44). The granules can be stained by the Grimelius and Masson-Fontana methods (Figure 3.45) and by immunohistochemical techniques for chromogranin, neuron-specific enolase, serotonin, and a variety of peptide hormones. Most primary carcinoid tumors have pursued a benign course, but rare examples have metastasized.[37]

Primitive Neuroectodermal Tumor

One primitive neuroectodermal tumor removed from a 30-year-old man has been described in the literature (Figure 3.46).[38] It was a 14-cm neoplasm composed predominantly of irregular masses of small undifferentiated cells with hyperchromatic nuclei and scanty cytoplasm (Figure 3.47). Occasional ependymal rosettes and tubular structures lined by several layers of primitive neuroectodermal cells were identified. Immunohistochemical staining for glial fibrillary acidic protein showed focal positivity of the tumor cells, confirming their neural nature. The tumor metastasized widely and was rapidly fatal. We have recently seen an additional similar tumor, which was composed predominantly of primitive neuroectodermal tissue in a 20-year-old man, as well as a mixed germ cell tumor with a minor primitive neuroectodermal component in a 17-year-old man (Figure 3.48); primitive neuroectodermal tissue predominated, however, in metastatic foci in the latter case. Four mixed germ cell tumors with components of primitive neuroectodermal tumor have recently been described in abstract form.[39] These tumors must be differentiated from other small cell tumors of the testis and paratesticular tissue such as embryonal rhabdomyosarcoma and lymphoma. In cases in which diagnostic features such as neural tubules, glia, true rosettes, and pseudorosettes are absent, immunohistochemical staining may be helpful diagnostically.

Tumors of More Than One Histological Type (Mixed Germ Cell Tumors)

Approximately one third of germ cell tumors are composed of two or more of the tumor types described above (except for the spermatocytic seminoma).[40] The clinical presentations of patients with these mixed tumors do not differ appreciably from those of patients with pure germ cell tumors of nonseminomatous types. The ages of the patients generally parallel those of patients with embryonal carcinoma, with the average age in one series being 30 years.[41] As one might expect from the younger age of patients with embryonal carcinoma in general, mixed germ cell tumors with a predominant component of embryonal carcinoma occur an average of five years earlier than tumors with a predominant component of seminoma.[42]

Mixed germ cell tumors characteristically have a variegated appearance on gross inspection, reflecting the features of their various components. In most specimens, the components are intermixed in such a manner that they cannot be distinguished clearly on gross examination (Figures 3.49, 3.50), but in occasional cases, particularly those in which seminoma is present, it and the other component may form discrete masses, which may be adjacent to one another (Figure 3.51) or separated by testicular parenchyma.

The relative proportions of the various components in mixed germ cell tumors have varied in the literature. Many of the earlier studies were conducted before recognition of the yolk sac tumor and, therefore, did not classify the cases according to modern criteria. The most recent comprehensive analysis of the various components in mixed germ cell tumors was in a study from Denmark,[40] in which 26% of 352 tumors contained embryonal carcinoma and teratoma (teratocarcinoma) (Figure 3.52), 16% contained embryonal carcinoma and seminoma (Figures 3.53, 3.54), and 11% contained embryonal carcinoma, teratoma, and yolk sac tumor. A great variety of other combinations may be seen (Figures 3.55, 3.56). In the Danish study, the remaining tumors were composed of the following combinations in descending order of frequency: embryonal carcinoma, teratoma, and choriocarcinoma; seminoma, embryonal carcinoma, and teratoma; seminoma and teratoma; embryonal carcinoma and yolk sac tumor (Figures 3.57, 3.58); embryonal carcinoma, yolk sac tumor, teratoma, and choriocarcinoma; and embryonal carcinoma and choriocarcinoma. Various other combinations of these tumors were seen rarely. In another investigation, 40% of mixed germ cell tumors contained foci of yolk sac tumor.[21] Because of quantitative variations among types of germ cell neoplasia in mixed germ cell tumors, ranging from microscopic foci to grossly discernible components, the appropriate terminology for these tumors often creates a problem, which has not been addressed in the literature. For example, immature teratomas may contain scattered microscopic foci of embryonal carcinomatous or yolk sac epithelium. We designate such tumors as immature teratomas with embryonal or yolk sac elements unless either of these components forms a confluent lesion arbitrarily set as 0.3 cm in diameter. When the lesion attains that diameter, we diagnose immature teratoma with embryonal carcinoma or yolk sac tumor, reporting the size of either component.

In almost all the cases in which various subtypes of germ cell neoplasia coexist, they form discrete foci that are either grossly discernible or are haphazardly distributed on microscopic examination of the tumor. In occasional cases, however, such components are diffusely intermixed in a more orderly manner throughout the specimen in distinctive patterns. A rare mixed germ cell tumor has embryonal carcinoma, yolk sac tumor, and chorionic elements distributed more or less uniformly throughout the specimen. Sometimes a distinctive necklace pattern with yolk sac elements wrapped around groups of embryonal carcinoma cells is encountered. These tumors have been referred to as "diffuse embryomas" (Figures 3.59 to 3.63).[43]

Perhaps the most common problem in the microscopic interpretation of mixed germ cell tumors involves the recognition of yolk sac elements within them, since such elements may simulate both embryonal carcinoma and seminoma in their growth patterns and cytological features. In general, yolk sac elements grow in a reticular pattern, which is rare or absent in other forms of germ cell tumor. However, papillae may be seen in both yolk sac tumors and embryonal carcinomas and a solid pattern may be seen in these two tumors as well as in seminoma. The cells of the yolk sac tumor, however, are generally smaller and less pleomorphic and have clearer cytoplasm than those of the embryonal carcinoma. In the distinction of yolk sac tumor from seminoma, a helpful clue is the presence of small glandular formations or slitlike spaces in the otherwise solid areas of yolk sac tumors and a lack of a sprinkling of lymphocytes within the tumor, a characteristic feature of seminomas. The use of AFP stains is helpful in identifying yolk sac elements in problematic cases.

Mixed germ cell tumors may metastasize in a variety of forms, including mature teratoma. In general, these tumors are less malignant than embryonal carcinomas. Like the latter, they are curable in a high proportion of cases by surgical removal with or without combination chemotherapy.

Occult Testicular Germ Cell Tumors

Five percent to 10% of patients with testicular germ cell tumors present with clinically normal testes and symptoms referable to extratesticular disease, which may involve retroperitoneal lymph nodes, mediastinal lymph nodes, distant organs, or a combination of these sites.[44] A variety of lesions may be encountered in the testis in such cases.[45,46] The testis may contain an invasive tumor that was not detectable clinically (Figures 3.64, 3.65), intratubular germ cell neoplasia, or in some cases only a scar (Figure 3.66).[46–52] Azzopardi and associates[46] described the cases of 17 young men who died with metastatic choriocarcinoma (eight cases), embryonal carcinoma (five cases), choriocarcinoma and embryonal carcinoma (three cases), and embryonal carcinoma and teratoma (one case), and had fibrous scars in their testes on gross examination. The scars were typically irregular (Figure 3.66), but were more or less well defined. On microscopic examination, ghost remnants of hyalinized seminiferous tubules were often present within the scars. There was only a scar in nine of the 17 cases, but an epidermoid cyst was also present in four cases and other teratomatous elements were present in four additional cases (Figure 3.67). A distinctive feature in the majority of the cases was the presence of oval or round nests of necrotic tissue containing hematoxylin-staining deposits, indicating the presence of necrotic intratubular embryonal carcinoma. Other findings were intratubular seminoma, necrotic seminoma, and intratubular germ cell neoplasia, unclassified (see Chapter 4). Subsequently, a somewhat similar phenomenon was described in cases of metastatic seminoma, except that the intratubular hematoxyphilic deposits seen in cases of retrogressed nonseminomatous tumors were not observed.[53]

Germ Cell Tumors After Chemotherapy

Metastatic germ cell tumors examined after the administration of chemotherapeutic agents may be found to contain viable-appearing tumor, necrotic tumor (Figure 3.68), replacement of tumor by scar tissue, and tumor tissue showing a higher degree of maturity then the primary testicular tumor (Figures 3.69 to 3.71). This "maturation" of tumor after chemotherapy is believed to be due to a failure of the more mature elements of the tumor to respond to treatment rather than true maturation of immature elements. Evidence favoring the former explanation is the finding of similar mature elements in the primary tumor in almost all of the cases in which they were found in the metastatic deposits after treatment.[54–57] The prognosis after metastatic foci with a teratomatous appearance have been surgically excised is generally favorable. Malignant tumors such as rhabdomyosarcoma, squamous cell carcinoma, and mucinous adenocarcinoma may arise in metastatic testicular germ cell tumors after treatment,[34,58–60] as may the unusual cystic lesions that resemble choriocarcinoma referred to earlier (see page 41).[29]

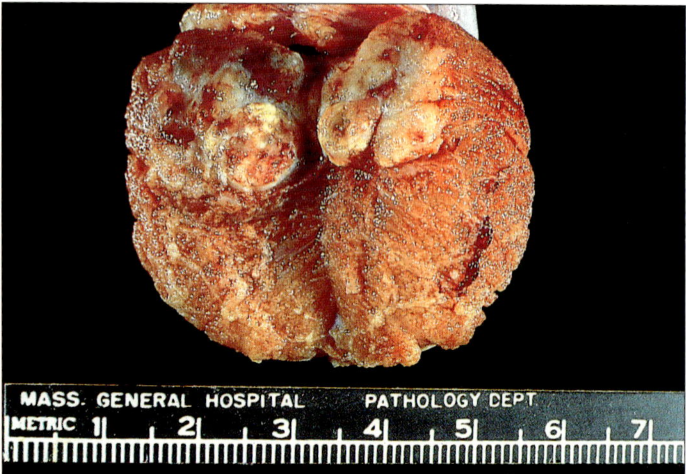

Figure 3.1 Embryonal carcinoma. The neoplastic tissue contains foci of necrosis and hemorrhage.

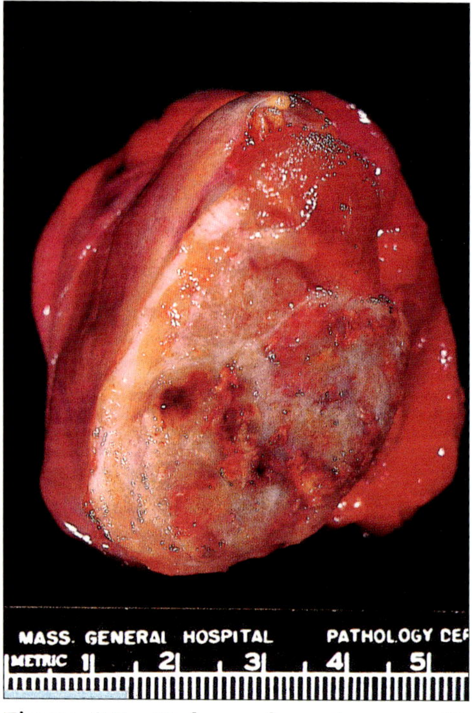

Figure 3.2 Embryonal carcinoma with extensive fibrosis, necrosis, and hemorrhage.

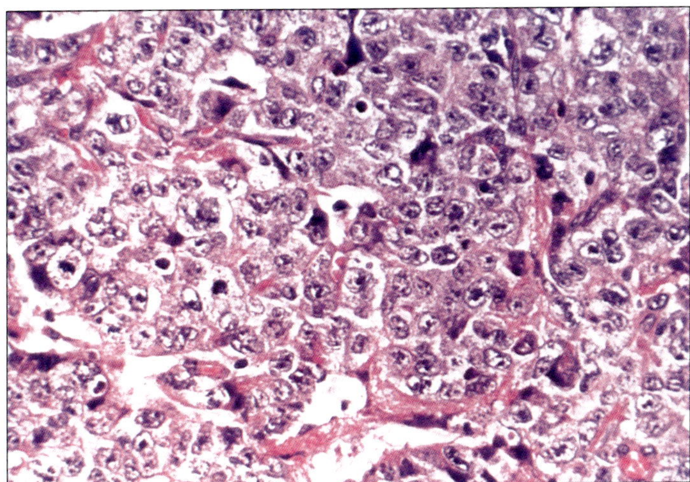

Figure 3.3 Embryonal carcinoma. The tumor cells are arranged diffusely and contain granular, amphophilic cytoplasm, and slightly irregular nuclei with prominent nucleoli.

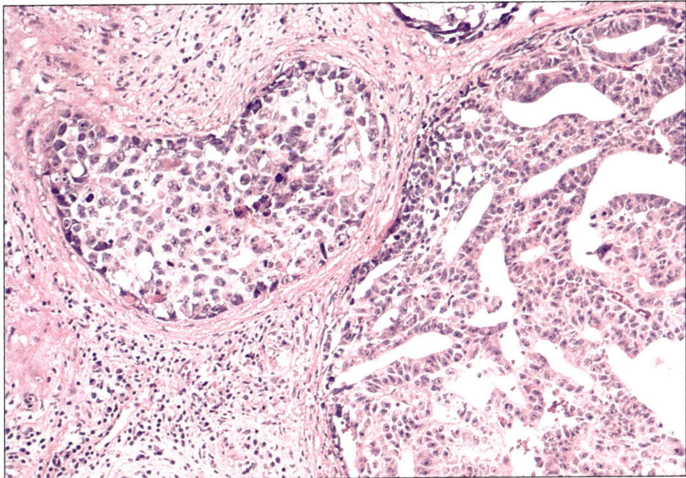

Figure 3.4 Embryonal carcinoma. The tumor has a glandular pattern in the right portion of the picture and fills a tubule in the left portion.

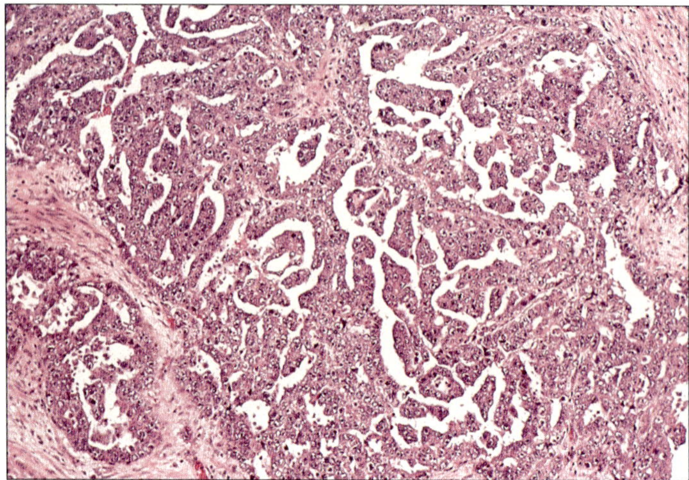

Figure 3.5 Embryonal carcinoma. The tumor has a papillary pattern.

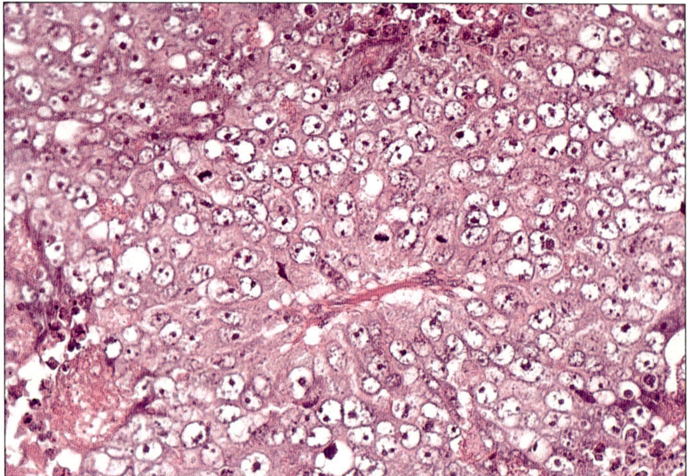

Figure 3.6 Embryonal carcinoma. The nuclei are very large and clear and contain prominent nucleoli. Several mitotic figures are present.

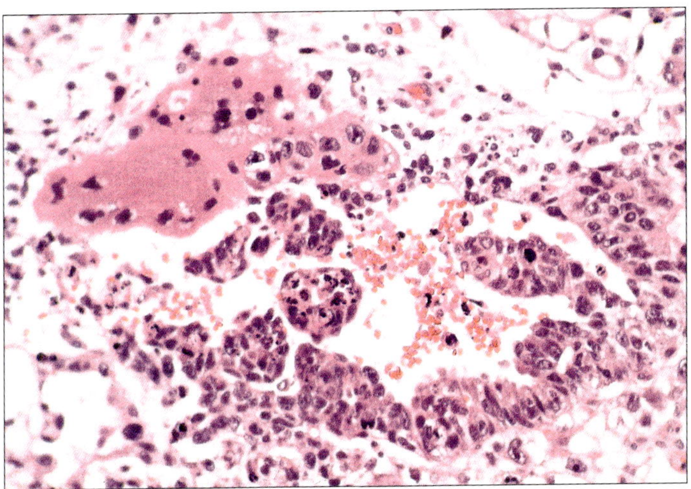

Figure 3.7 Embryonal carcinoma with syncytiotrophoblast cells.

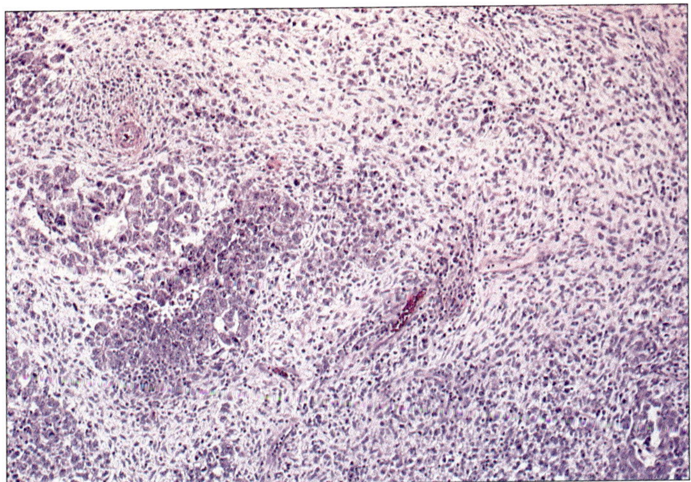

Figure 3.8 Embryonal carcinoma. Islands of embryonal carcinoma cells are separated by a highly cellular mesenchyme.

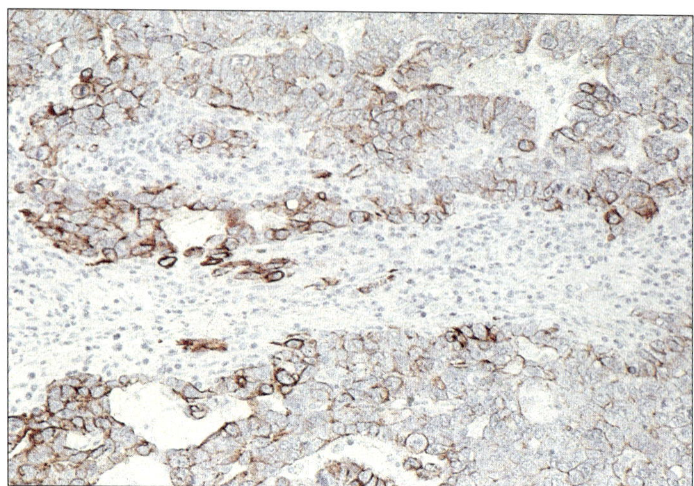

Figure 3.9 Embryonal carcinoma. The tumor cells are stained immunohistochemically for cytokeratin.

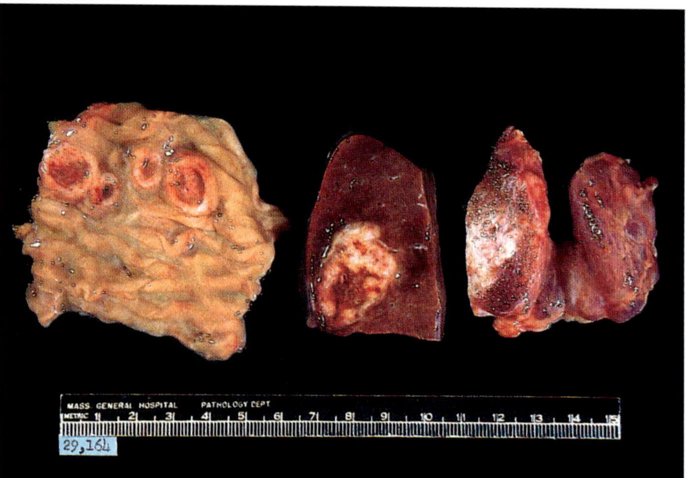

Figure 3.10 Embryonal carcinoma. The mucosal surface of the small intestine and sectioned surfaces of the liver and thyroid gland are the sites of hematogenous metastases.

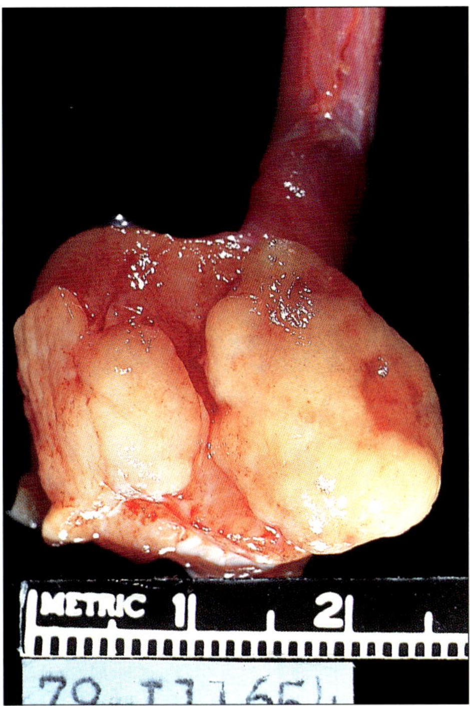

Figure 3.11 Yolk sac tumor of infantile testis. The neoplastic tissue has a homogenous, pale yellow, bulging appearance.

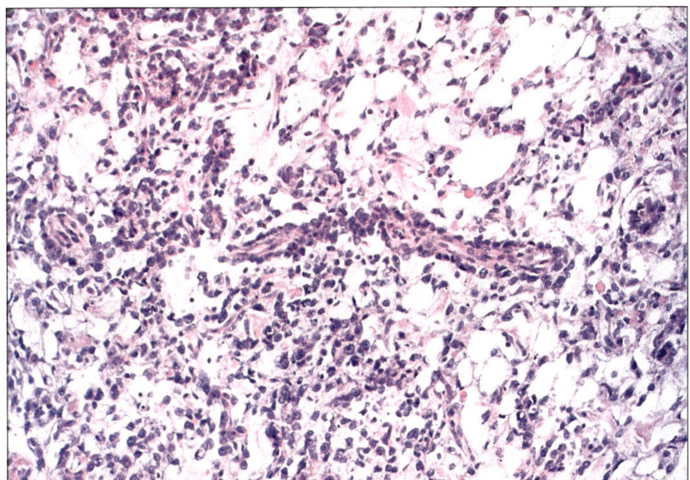

Figure 3.12 Yolk sac tumor. The neoplastic cells are arranged in a reticular pattern. Cross and longitudinal sections of several Schiller-Duval bodies are visible.

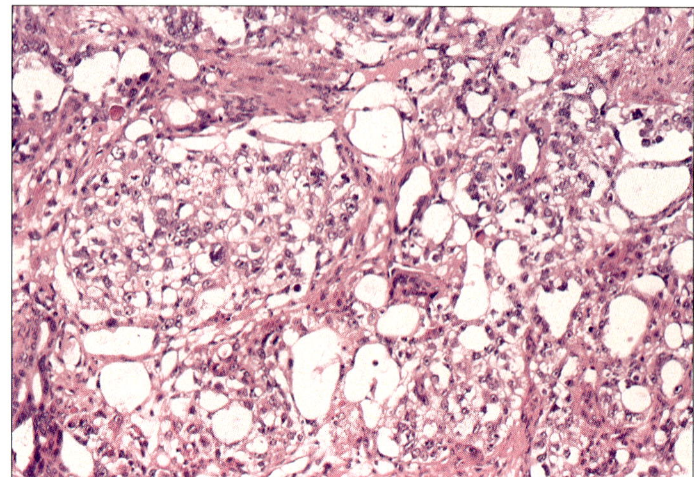

Figure 3.13 Yolk sac tumor. The tumor has a microcystic pattern.

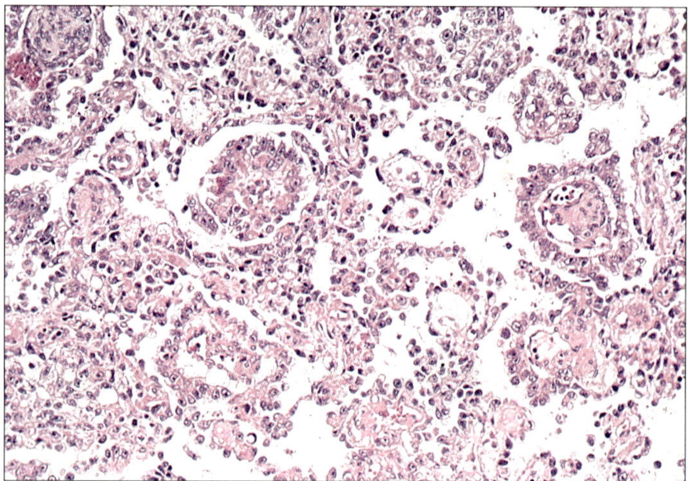

Figure 3.14 Yolk sac tumor. Numerous Schiller-Duval bodies are present.

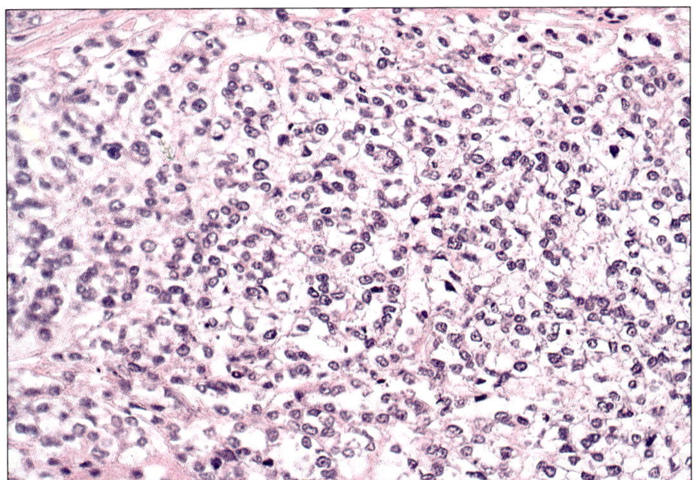

Figure 3.15 Yolk sac tumor. The neoplastic cells are growing in a solid pattern and have clear cytoplasm and relatively uniform nuclei, simulating the appearance of a seminoma.

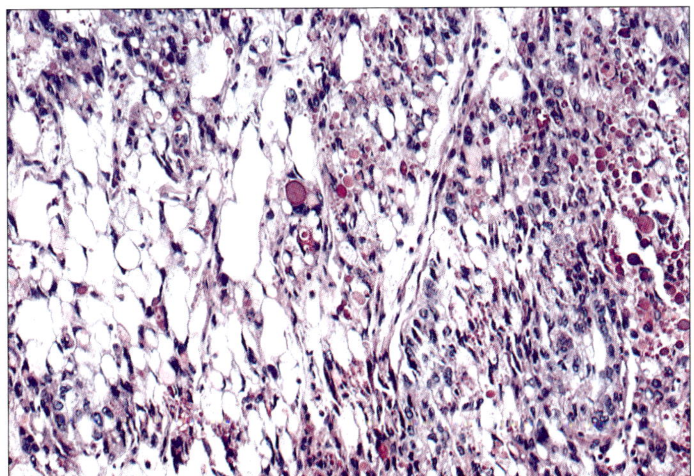

Figure 3.16 Yolk sac tumor. Many of the neoplastic cells have a vacuolated appearance, simulating a liposarcoma. Numerous hyaline bodies are visible.

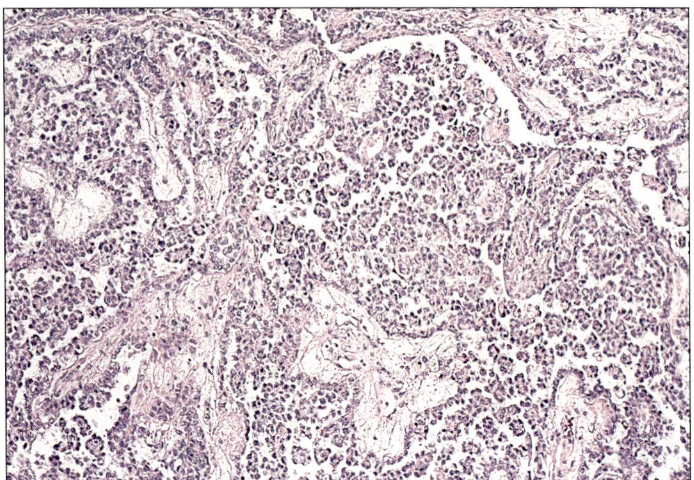

Figure 3.17 Yolk sac tumor. The neoplastic cells are growing in a papillary pattern.

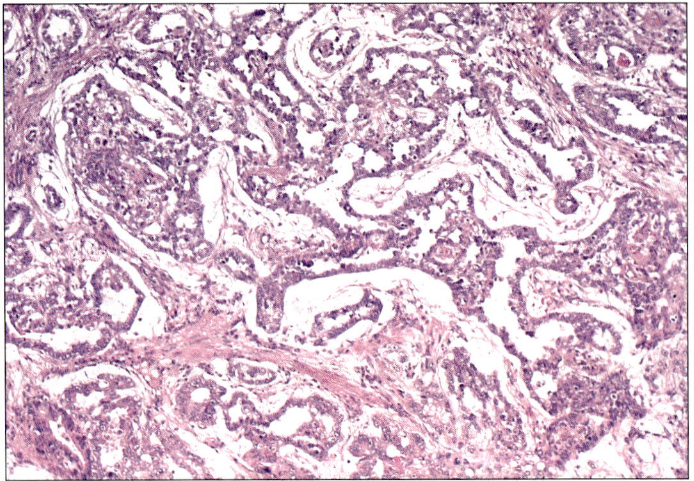

Figure 3.18 Yolk sac tumor. The tumor cells have a festoon pattern.

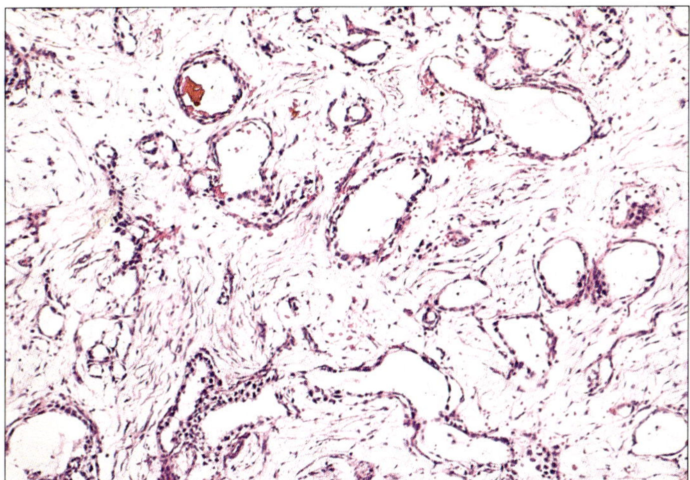

Figure 3.19 Yolk sac tumor. The neoplastic cells have a polyvesicular vitelline pattern, with the vesicles separated by hypocellular mesenchyme. One vesicle in the right upper portion of the picture has an eccentric constriction, recapitulating the division of the primary yolk sac (larger component) into the secondary yolk sac (smaller component).

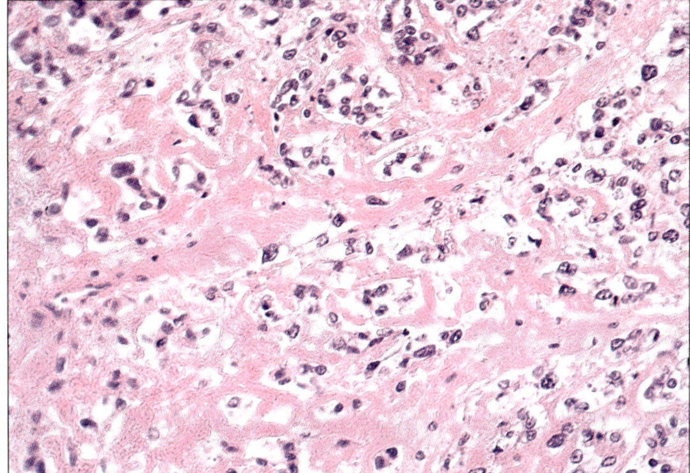

Figure 3.20 Yolk sac tumor with parietal pattern. Clusters of neoplastic cells are separated by abundant, eosinophilic basement membrane material.

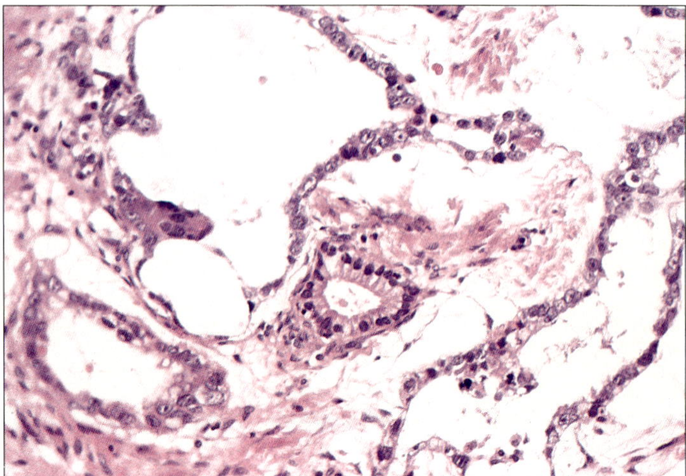

Figure 3.21 Yolk sac tumor. A small gland lined by mucinous epithelium is present in the center.

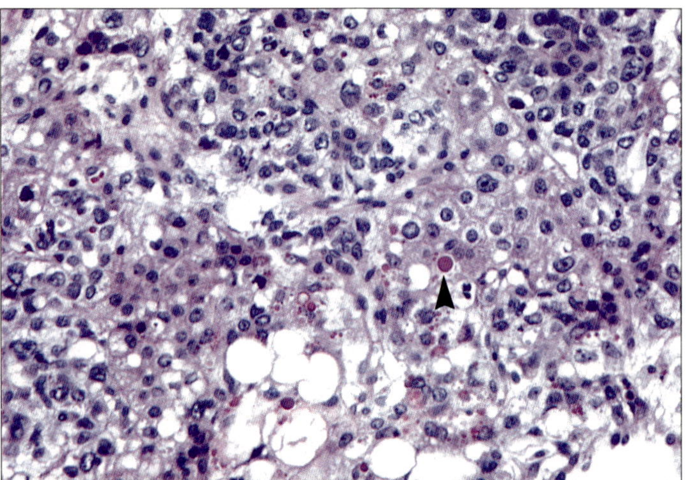

Figure 3.22 Yolk sac tumor. A nest of cells resembling hepatocytes and containing hyaline bodies (arrow) is present to the right of the center.

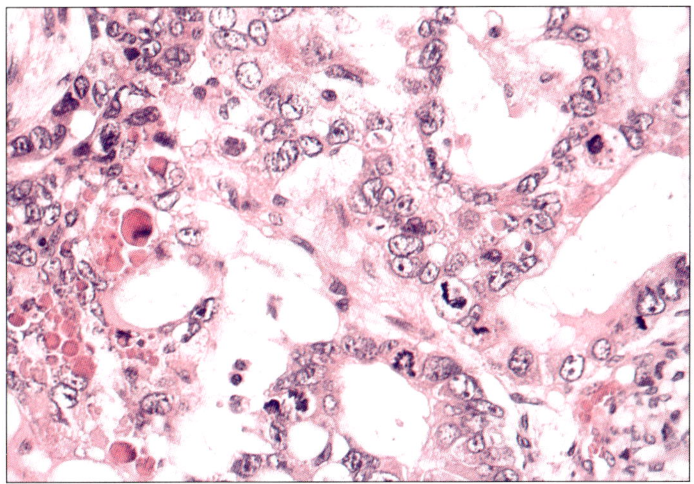

Figure 3.23 Yolk sac tumor. The tumor cells are forming glandular structures. The cells have abundant amphophilic cytoplasm and large atypical nuclei showing atypical mitotic activity. Numerous hyaline bodies are visible.

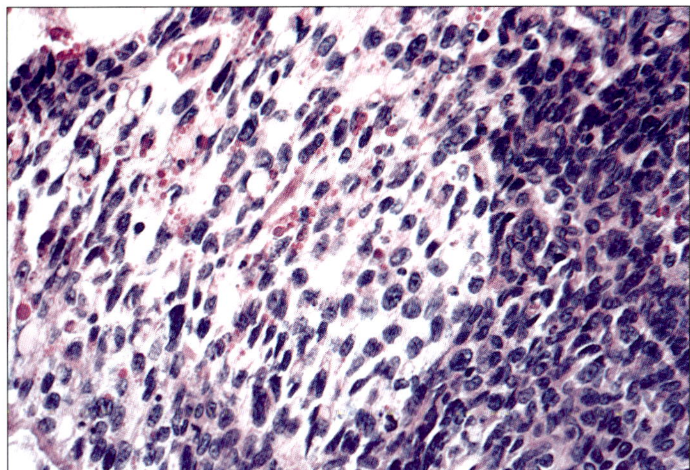

Figure 3.24 Yolk sac tumor. Closely packed cells with scanty cytoplasm and hyperchromatic nuclei are present in the right portion of the picture. Hyaline bodies are also visible.

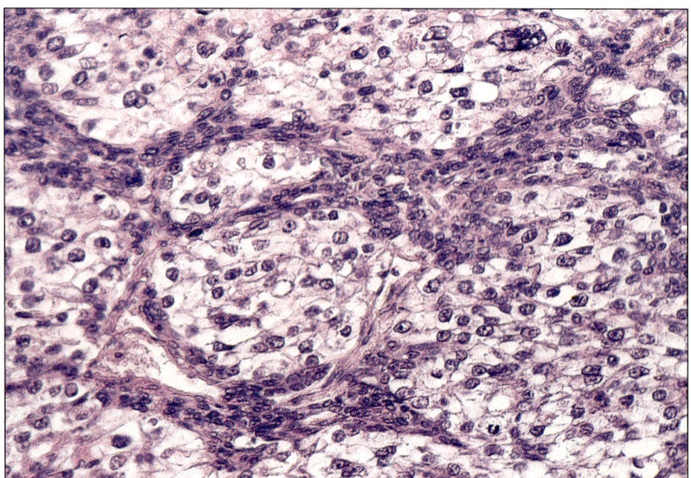

Figure 3.25 Yolk sac tumor. The neoplastic cells have a solid pattern and are large and polyhedral with abundant clear cytoplasm, creating a resemblance to renal cell carcinoma.

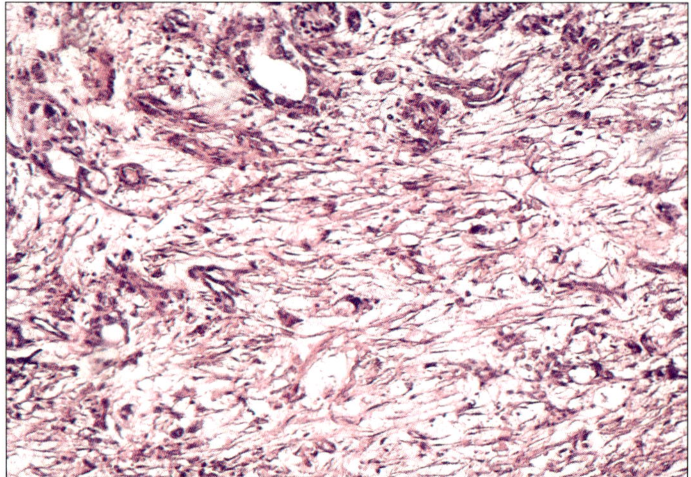

Figure 3.26 Yolk sac tumor. The neoplastic cells are separated by abundant myxoid stroma.

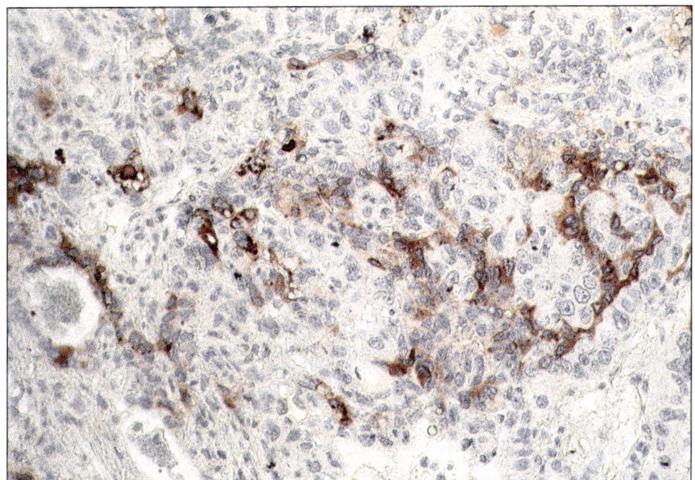

Figure 3.27 Yolk sac tumor. Many of the cells are stained immunohistochemically for α-fetoprotein.

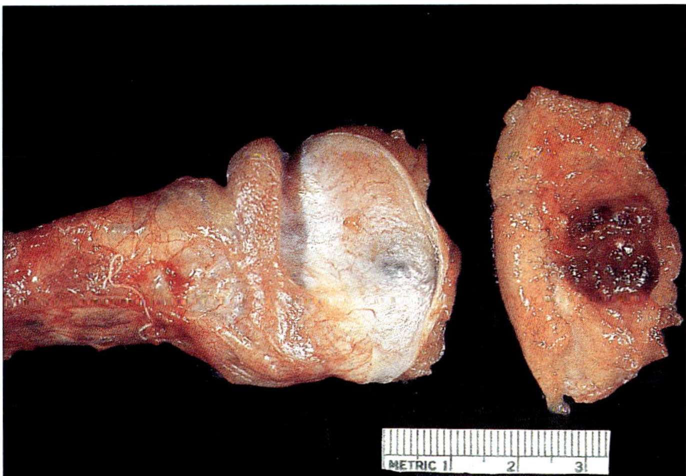

Figure 3.28 Choriocarcinoma. The tumor is small and diffusely hemorrhagic. A blue protuberance of the tumor is seen on the tunica albuginea.

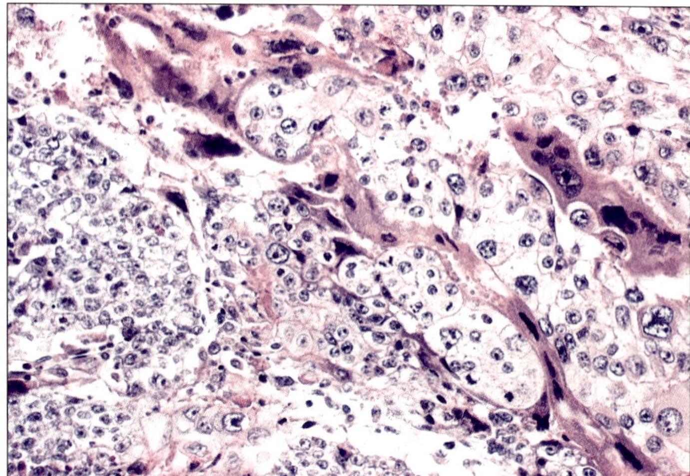

Figure 3.29 Choriocarcinoma. Groups of cells resembling cytotrophoblast (far left) and intermediate trophoblast (center) are associated with syncytiotrophoblast cells, which have multiple nuclei and abundant eosinophilic cytoplasm.

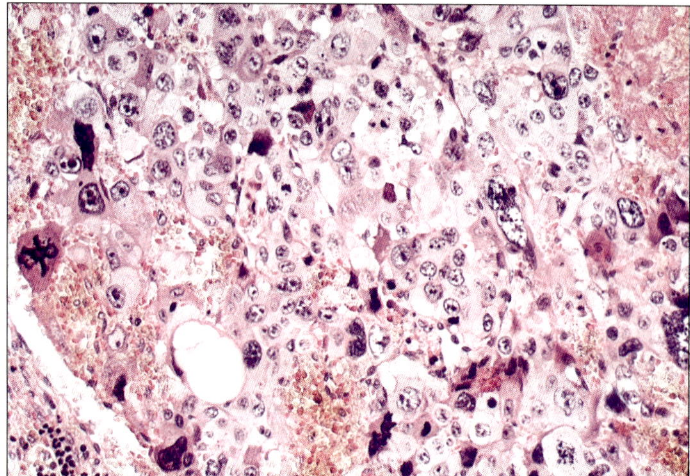

Figure 3.30 Choriocarcinoma. In this tumor, the trophoblast cells are poorly differentiated and not as clearly separable into the various subtypes illustrated in the previous figure.

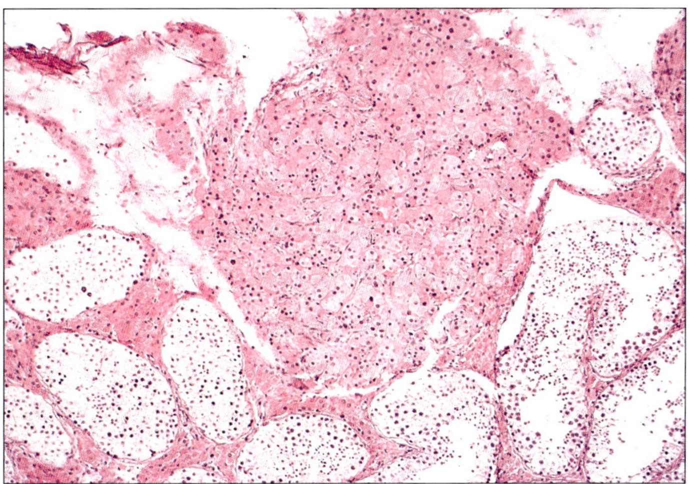

Figure 3.31 Leydig cell hyperplasia in association with choriocarcinoma.

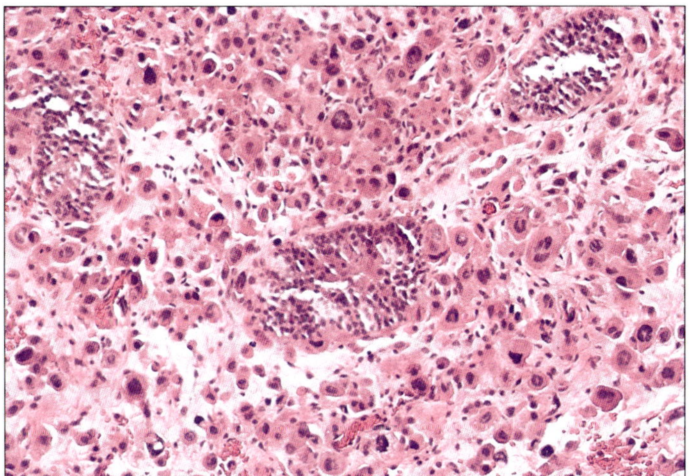

Figure 3.32 Placental site trophoblastic tumor. The tumor is composed of cells resembling the intermediate trophoblast cells of the placental site. The tumor surrounds immature testicular tubules.

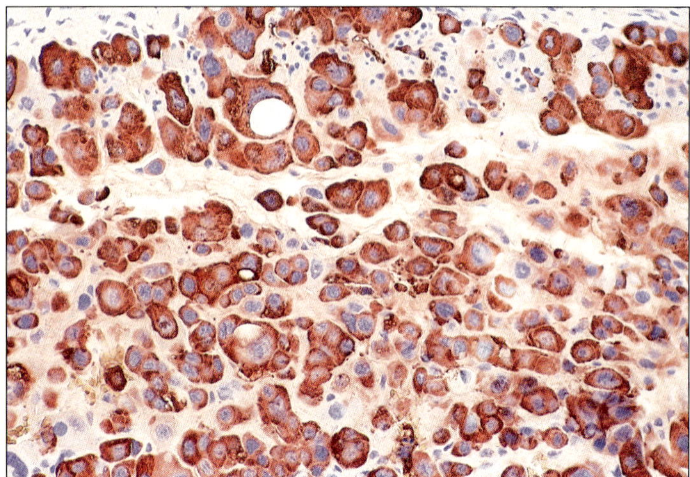

Figure 3.33 Placental site trophoblastic tumor. The tumor cells in the case illustrated in the previous figure are stained immunohistochemically for placental lactogen.

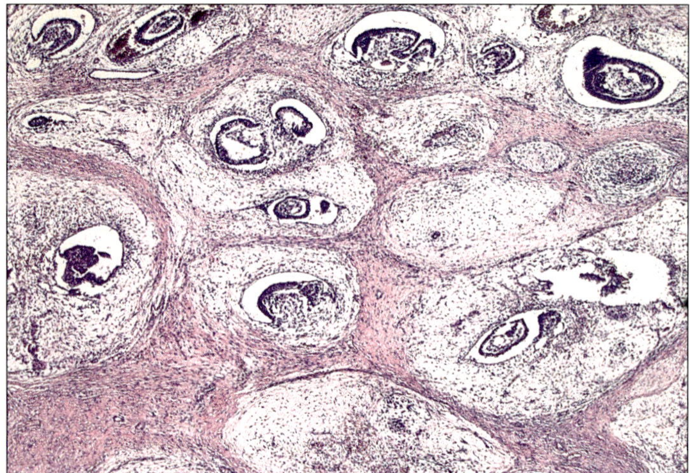

Figure 3.34 Polyembryoma. Numerous embryoid bodies are present, consisting of amniotic cavity, germ disc, yolk sac, and extraembryonic mesenchyme.

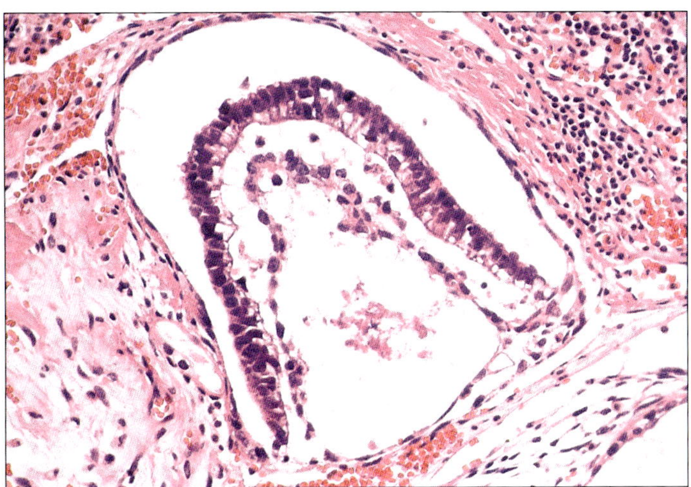

Figure 3.35 Polyembryoma. An embryoid body consists of amniotic sac, germ disc, and yolk sac in the center.

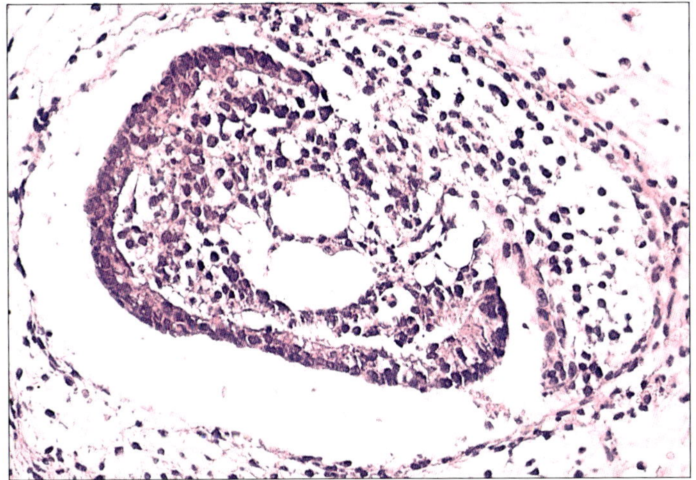

Figure 3.36 Polyembryoma. An embryoid body consists of an amniotic cavity (far left and below), germ disc, and yolk sac (center).

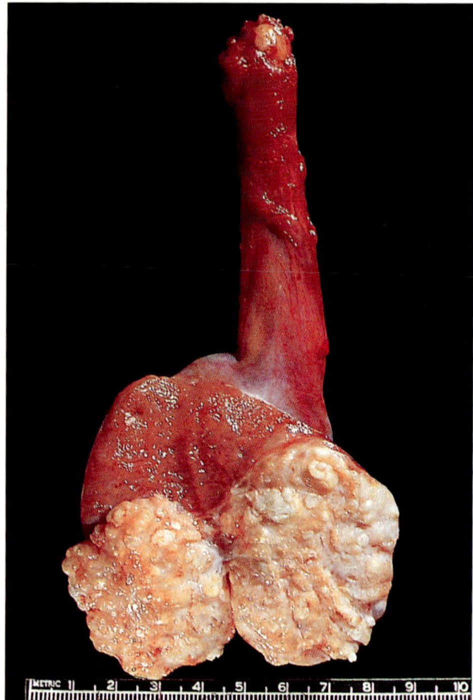

Figure 3.37 Mature teratoma. The tumor is predominantly solid.

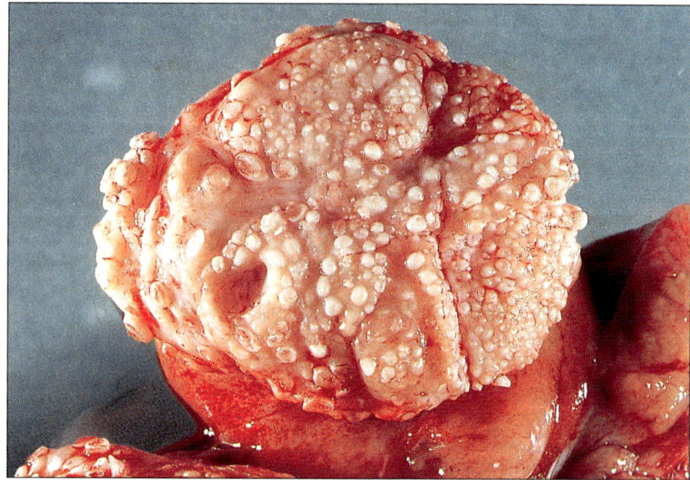

Figure 3.38 Mature teratoma. The numerous nodules were composed of cysts lined by squamous epithelium and filled with keratinous material.

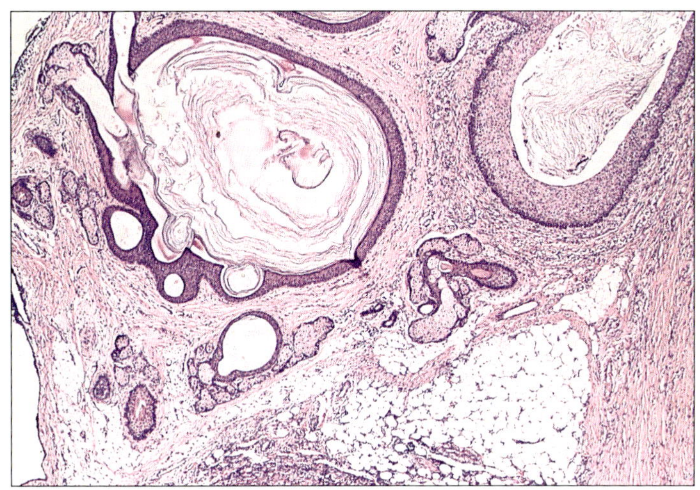

Figure 3.39 Mature teratoma. Cysts lined by squamous epithelium and filled with keratin, sebaceous glands, and adipose tissue are present.

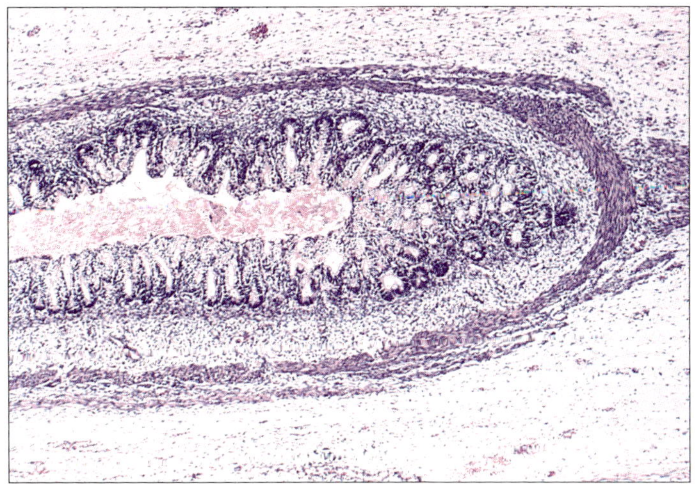

Figure 3.40 Mature teratoma. The wall of an intestinal tube is composed of mucosa, submucosa, and muscularis.

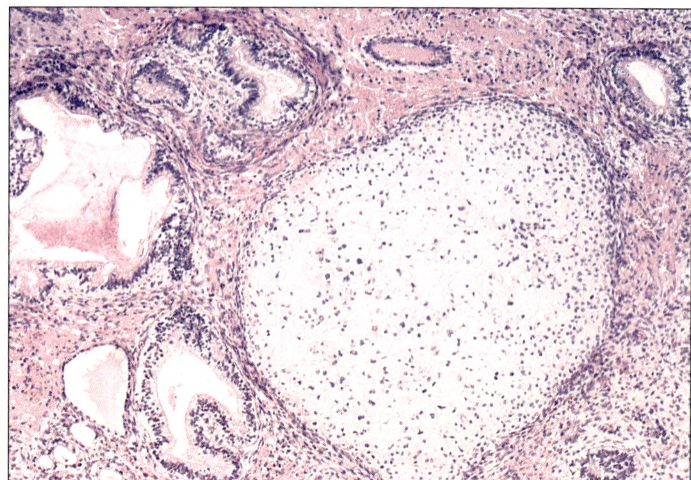

Figure 3.41 Teratoma, immature. Glands lined by slightly immature intestinal epithelium and an island of cellular cartilage are present.

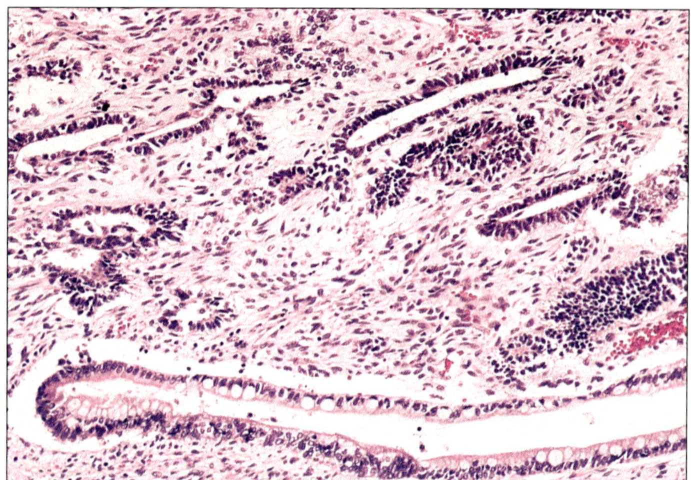

Figure 3.42 Teratoma, immature. In addition to a tubule lined by intestinal-type epithelium, multiple, slightly immature, neuroectodermal tubules are present.

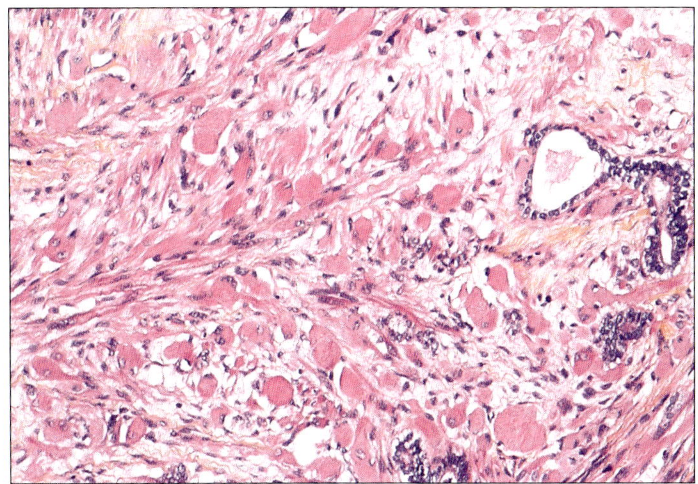

Figure 3.43 Rhabdyomyosarcoma arising in teratoma.

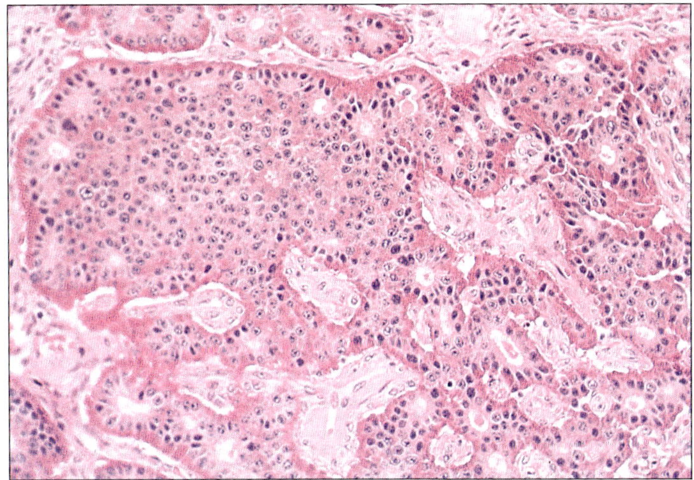

Figure 3.44 Carcinoid, insular type. The tumor is composed of islands and anastomosing trabeculae of cells with central round nuclei containing coarse chromatin. Numerous red argentaffin granules are present within the cytoplasm of the cells, particularly along the periphery of the nests and trabeculae.

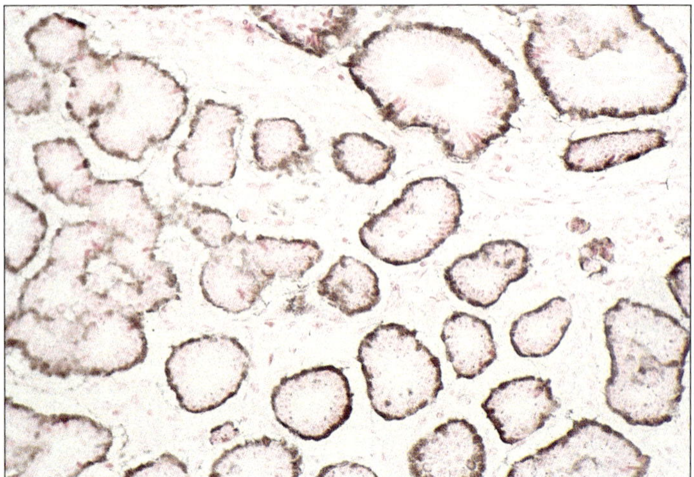

Figure 3.45 Carcinoid, insular type. The argentaffin cells are stained brownish-black by the Masson-Fontana technique.

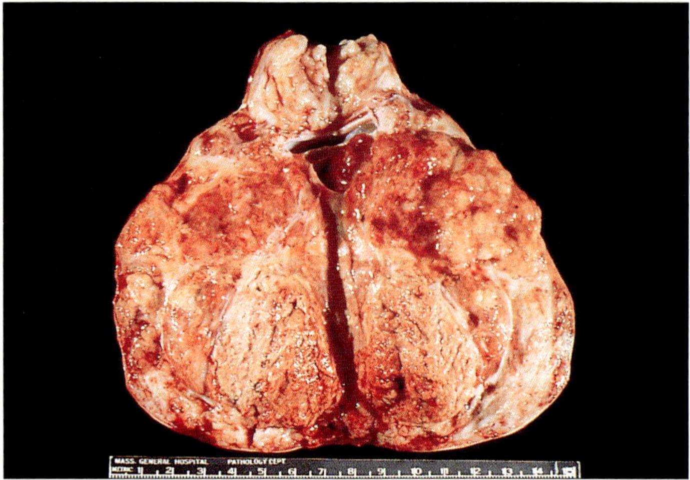

Figure 3.46 Primitive neuroectodermal tumor. The neoplastic tissue appears soft and contains foci of necrosis and hemorrhage.

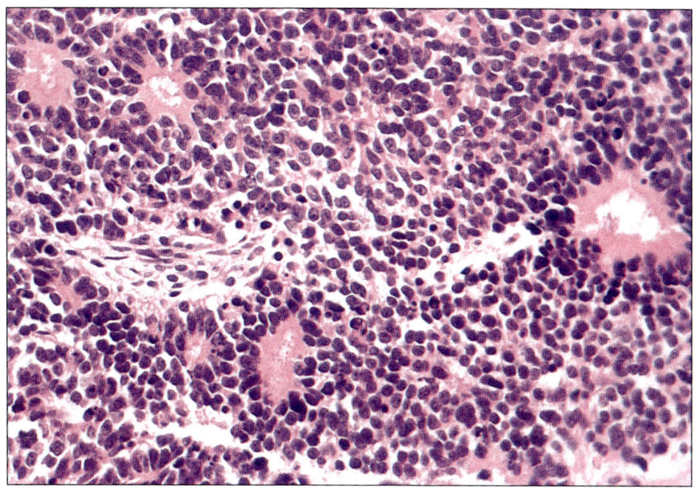

Figure 3.47 Primitive neuroectodermal tumor. True rosettes are present within an otherwise solid area of primitive neuroectodermal cells.

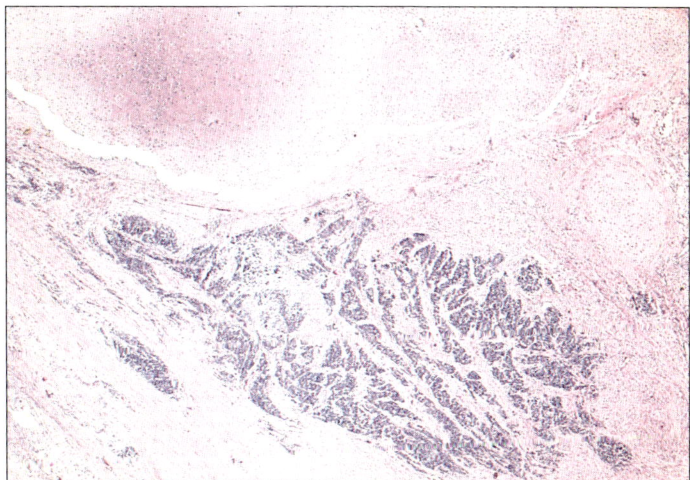

Figure 3.48 Mixed germ cell tumor. A small focus of primitive neuroectodermal tumor is present. Cartilage is present at the top and right.

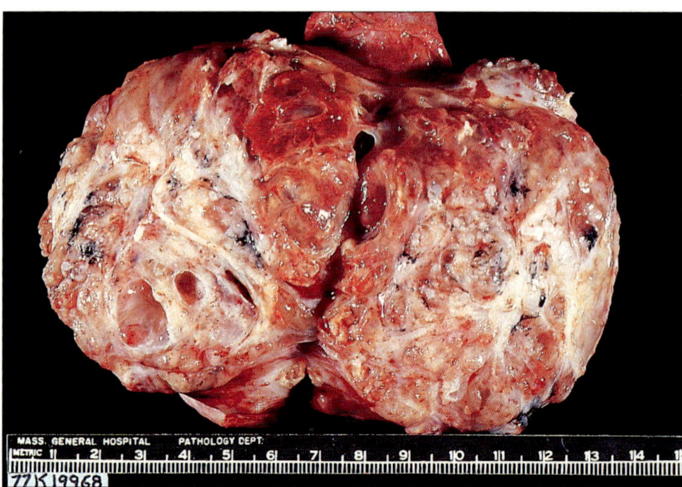

Figure 3.49 Mixed germ cell tumor. This tumor is a mixture of teratoma and embryonal carcinoma (teratocarcinoma). The embryonal carcinoma is suggested by the necrotic and hemorrhagic tissue. The presence of cysts and small foci of black discoloration (pigmented retinal tissue) is evidence of a teratomatous component.

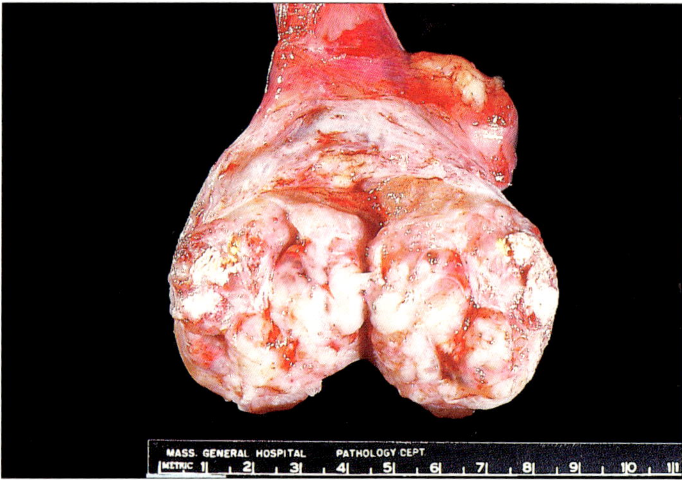

Figure 3.50 Mixed germ cell tumor. In this tumor, seminoma and teratoma are intimately admixed and cannot be clearly distinguished on gross examination.

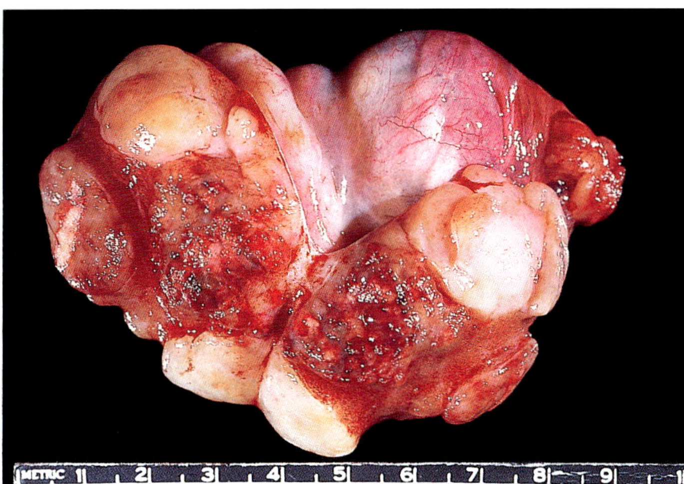

Figure 3.51 Mixed germ cell tumor. The neoplasm is composed of two nodules of soft, uniform, cream-colored seminoma separated by focally necrotic and hemorrhagic embryonal carcinoma.

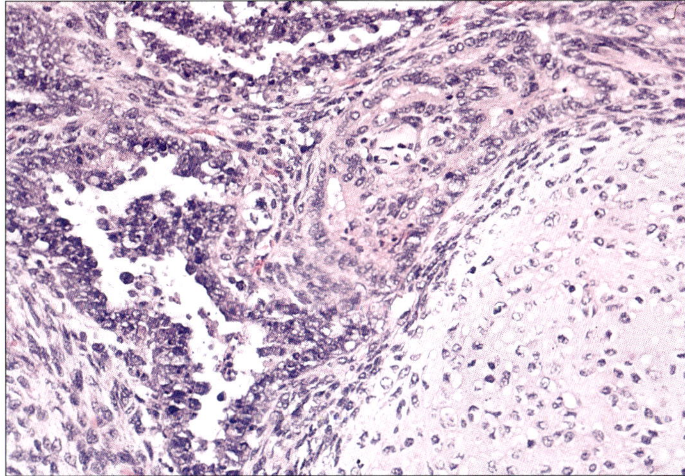

Figure 3.52 Embryonal carcinoma and teratoma (teratocarcinoma). Embryonal carcinoma forming glands is present adjacent to slightly immature cartilage.

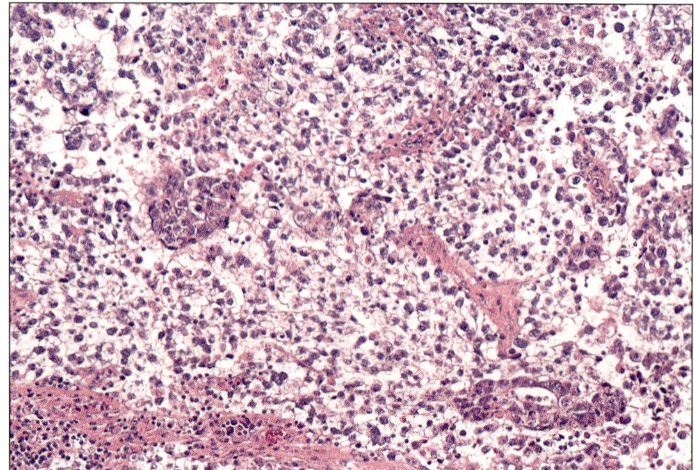

Figure 3.53 Embryonal carcinoma and seminoma. Several islands of embryonal carcinoma lie within a seminoma.

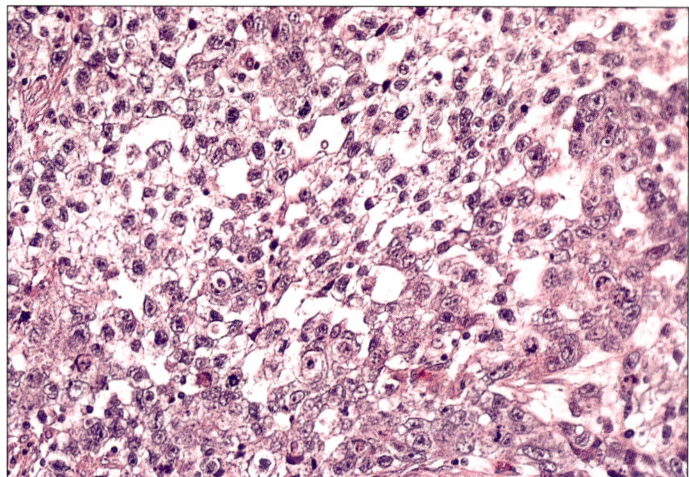

Figure 3.54 Embryonal carcinoma and seminoma. The seminoma cells are smaller and have clearer cytoplasm and smaller nuclei than the embryonal carcinoma cells.

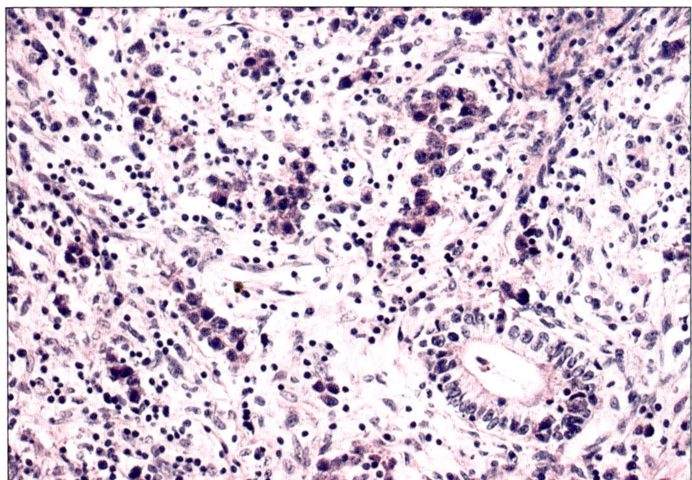

Figure 3.55 Seminoma and teratoma. Clusters of seminoma cells lie in a loose stroma infiltrated by lymphocytes. A teratomatous, probably endodermal gland is also present.

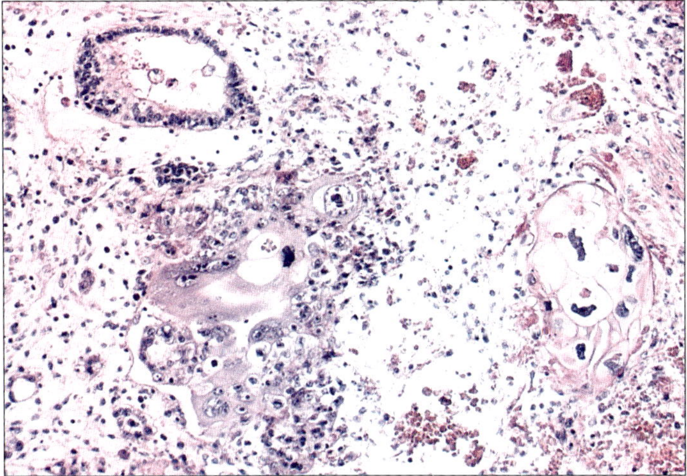

Figure 3.56 Choriocarcinoma and teratoma. A small focus of choriocarcinoma composed predominantly of syncytiotrophoblast cells accompanies a teratomatous gland and a teratomatous island of bizarre squamous cells (right).

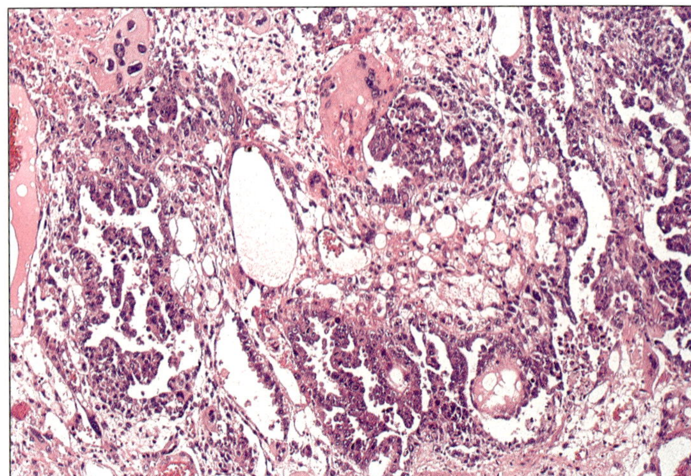

Figure 3.57 Embryonal carcinoma with syncytiotrophoblast cells and yolk sac tumor. The embryonal carcinoma has papillary and glandular patterns. The yolk sac tumor is represented by a vacuolated area just to the right of center.

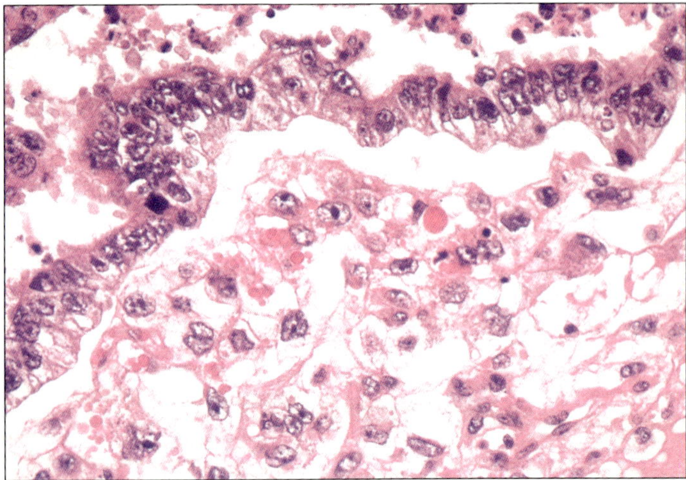

Figure 3.58 Embryonal carcinoma and yolk sac tumor. The yolk sac tumor cells have more abundant, clearer cytoplasm and contain hyaline bodies.

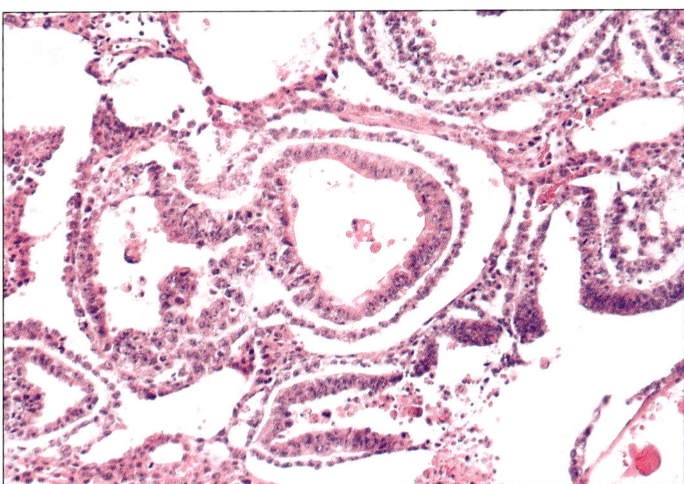

Figure 3.59 "Diffuse embryoma." The yolk sac elements are forming necklacelike structures surrounding circlets of much larger embryonal carcinoma cells.

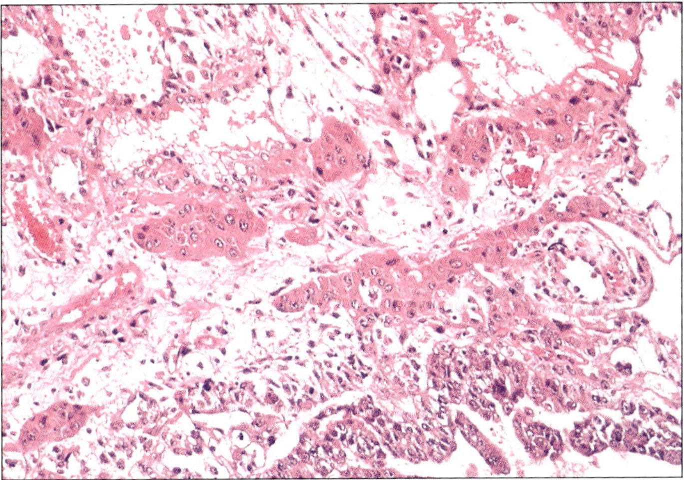

Figure 3.60 "Diffuse embryoma." Embryonal carcinoma is present at the bottom of the photomicrograph. Numerous islands of cells resembling hepatocytes are also illustrated.

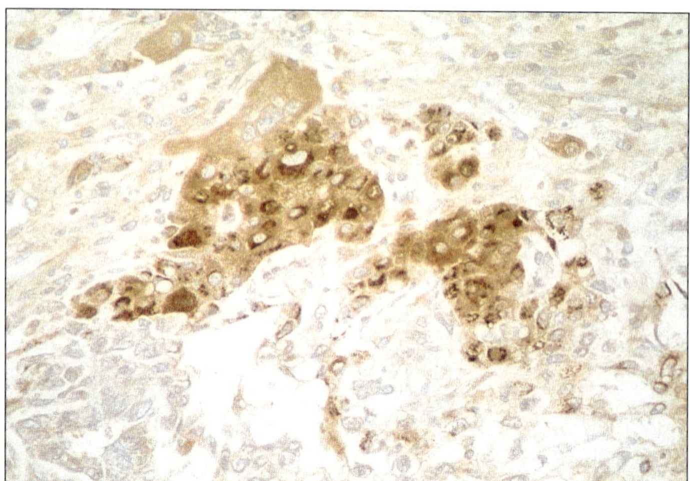

Figure 3.61 "Diffuse embryoma." The cells resembling hepatocytes are stained for α-fetoprotein.

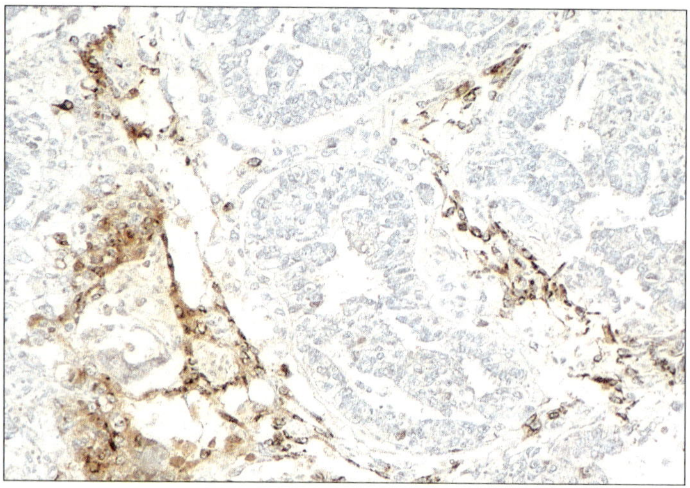

Figure 3.62 "Diffuse embryoma." The yolk sac component is stained for α-fetoprotein; the embryonal carcinoma is not stained.

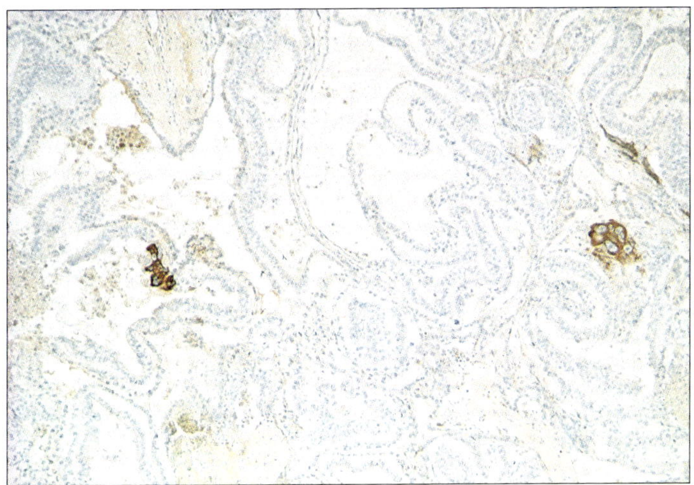

Figure 3.63 "Diffuse embryoma." Syncytiotrophoblast cells are stained immunohistochemically for chorionic gonadotropin.

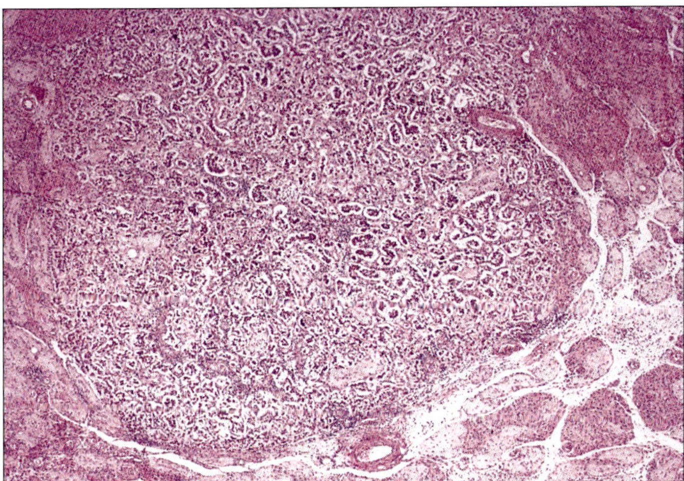

Figure 3.64 Seminoma, occult. This small tumor was associated with widespread metastases composed of embryonal carcinoma and choriocarcinoma.

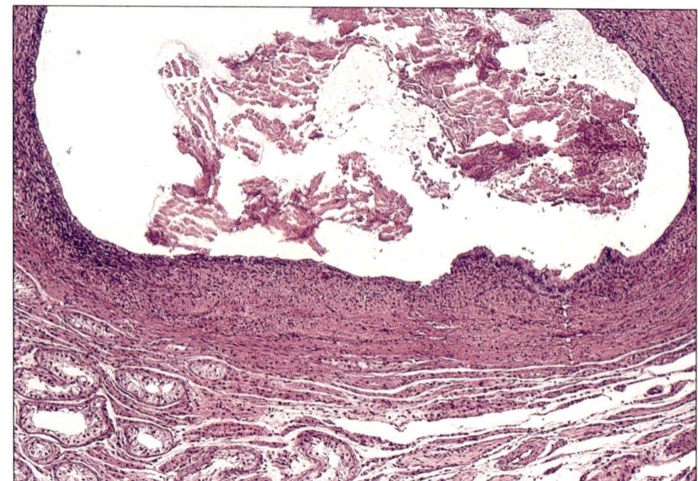

Figure 3.65 Teratoma, mature, occult. This patient had a retroperitoneal mass containing yolk sac tumor.

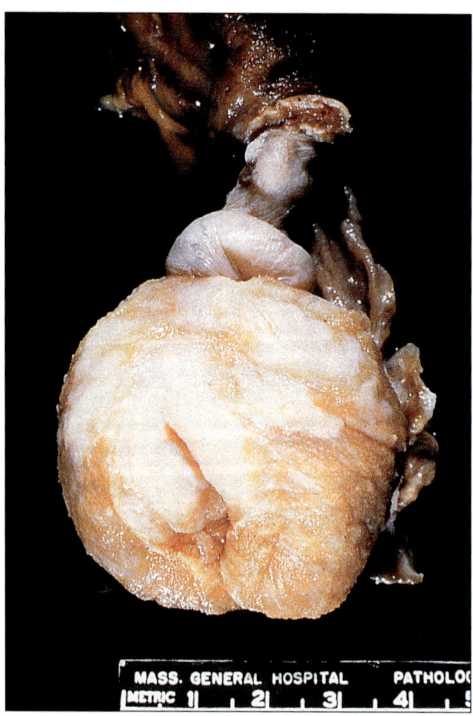

Figure 3.66 Retrogressed germ cell tumor. The tumor is represented by an irregular, white scar.

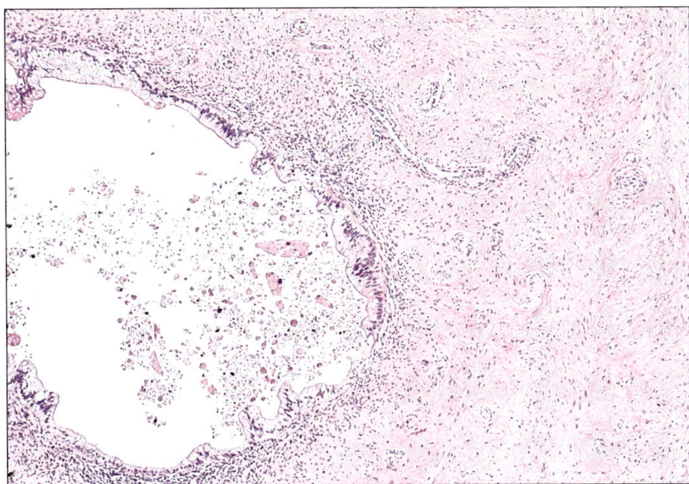

Figure 3.67 Retrogressed germ cell tumor. A teratomatous cyst lined by mucinous epithelium is present within a scar.

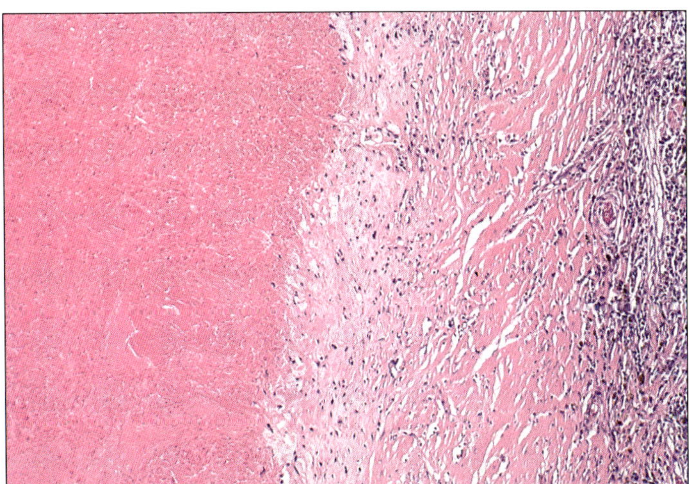

Figure 3.68 Germ cell tumor, metastatic, retroperitoneal, after chemotherapy. The tumor is diffusely necrotic and is surrounded by hyalinized scar tissue.

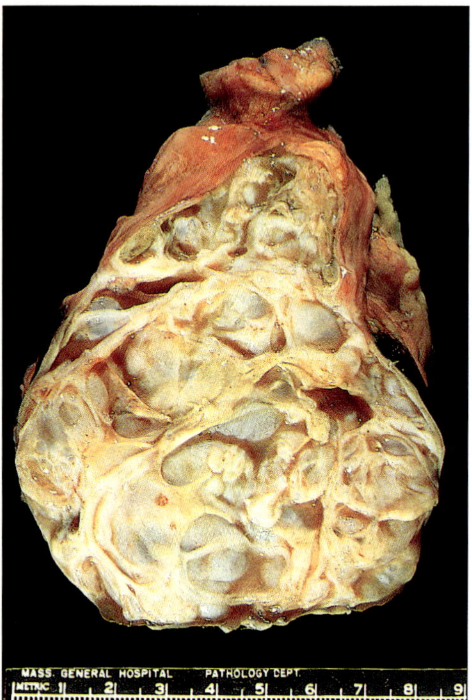

Figure 3.69 Germ cell tumor, metastatic, retroperitoneal, after chemotherapy. This tumor was a pure mature teratoma; the testicular tumor was embryonal carcinoma and teratoma.

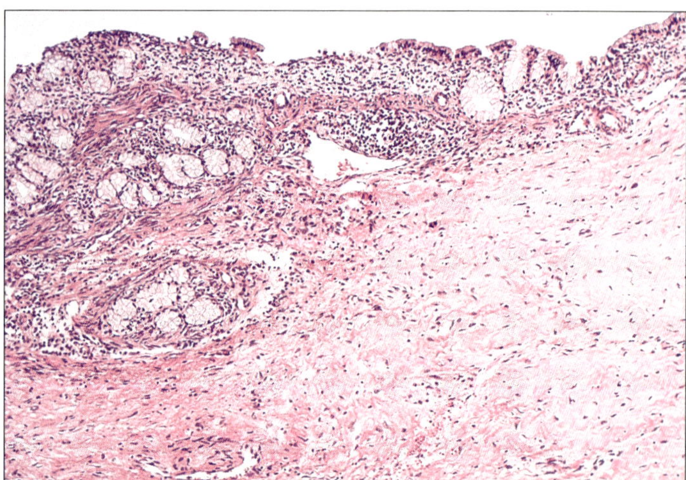

Figure 3.70 Germ cell tumor, metastatic, retroperitoneal, after chemotherapy. Cyst shown in Figure 3.69 is lined by epithelium with underlying glands resembling gastric mucosa.

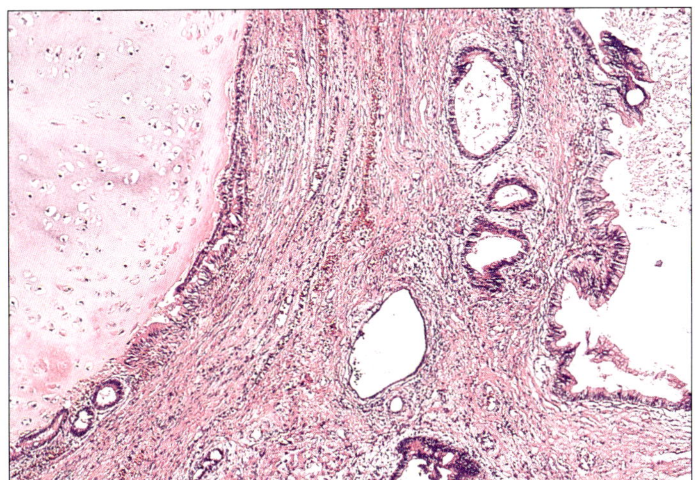

Figure 3.71 Germ cell tumor, metastatic, retroperitoneal, after chemotherapy. The tumor is a mature teratoma containing mucinous glands and cysts and an island of cartilage. The testicular tumor was represented by a scar containing a few teratomatous foci.

References

1. Mostofi FK. Classification of tumors of testis. *Ann Clin Lab Sci* 9:455–461, 1979.
2. Mostofi FK, Price EB Jr. *Atlas of Tumor Pathology,* Second Series, Fascicle 8. *Tumors of the Male Genital System*. Washington, DC, Armed Forces Institute of Pathology, 1973.
3. Friedman M, DiRienzo AJ. Trophocarcinoma (embryonal carcinoma) of the testis: Factors influencing radiation and surgical treatment. *Cancer* 16:868–884, 1963.
4. Marin-Padilla M. Histopathology of the embryonal carcinoma of the testis: Embryological evaluation. *Arch Pathol Lab Med* 85:614–622, 1968.
5. Pierce GB, Abell MR. Embryonal carcinoma of the testis. *Pathol Annu* 5:27–60, 1970.
6. Vugrin D, Chen A, Feigl P, Laszlo J. Embryonal carcinoma of the testis. *Cancer* 61:2348–2352, 1988.
7. Battifora H, Sheibani K, Tubbs RR, et al. Antikeratin antibodies in tumor diagnosis. *Cancer* 54:843–848, 1984.
8. Miettinen M, Virtanen I, Talerman A. Intermediate filament proteins in human testis and testicular germ-cell lesions. *Int J Gynecol Pathol* 3:261–276, 1984.
9. Magner D, Campbell JS, Wiglesworth FW. Testicular adenocarcinoma with clear cells, occurring in infancy. *Cancer* 9:165–175, 1956.
10. Teoh TB, Steward JK, Willis RA. The distinctive adenocarcinoma of the infant's testis: An account of 15 cases. *J Pathol Bacteriol* 80:147–156, 1960.
11. Pierce GB, Bullock WK, Huntington RW Jr. Yolk sac tumors of the testis. *Cancer* 25:644–658, 1970.
12. Young PG, Mount BM, Foote FW Jr, Whitmore WF Jr. Embryonal adenocarcinoma in the prepubertal testis: A clinicopathologic study of 18 cases. *Cancer* 26:1065–1075, 1970.
13. Jeffs RD. Management of embryonal adenocarcinoma of the testis in childhood: An analysis of 164 cases. In: *Cancer in Childhood*, Godden JO, ed. New York, Plenum Press. 1973, pp 68–77.
14. Woodtli W, Hedinger C. Endodermal sinus tumor or orchioblastoma in children and adults. *Virchows Arch A* 364:93–110, 1974.
15. Wold LE, Kramer SA, Farrow GM. Testicular yolk sac and embryonal carcinomas in pediatric patients: Comparative immunohistochemical and clinicopathologic study. *Am J Clin Pathol* 81:427–435, 1984.
16. Kozakewich HPW, Rice E, Vawter CF, et al. Yolk sac tumor of the testis in children. *Lab Invest* 50:32A, 1984.
17. Griffin, GC, Raney RB Jr, Snyder H McC, et al. Yolk sac carcinoma of the testis in children. *J Urol* 137:954–957, 1987.

18. Kaplan GW, Cromie WC, Kelalis PP, et al. Prepubertal yolk sac testicular tumors: report of the testicular tumor registry. *J Urol* 140:1109–1112, 1988.
19. Talerman A. Yolk sac tumour associated with seminoma of the testis in adults. *Cancer* 33:1468–1473, 1974.
20. Talerman A. The incidence of yolk sac tumor (endodermal sinus tumor) elements in germ cell tumors of the testis in adults. *Cancer* 36:211–215, 1975.
21. Talerman A. Endodermal sinus (yolk sac) tumor elements in testicular germ-cell tumors in adults: Comparison of prospective and retrospective studies. *Cancer* 46:1213–1217, 1980.
22. Jacobsen GK, Jacobsen M. Possible liver cell differentiation in testicular germ cell tumours. *Histopathology* 7:537–548, 1983.
23. Eglen DE, Ulbright TM. The differential diagnosis of yolk sac tumor and seminoma: Usefulness of cytokeratin, alpha-fetoprotein, and alpha-l-antitrypsin immunoperoxidase reactions. *Am J Clin Pathol* 88:328–332, 1987.
24. Henry SC, Walsh PC, Rotner MB. Choriocarcinoma of the testis. *J Urol* 112:105–108, 1974.
25. Brigden ML, Sullivan LD, Comisarow RH. Case report: Stage C pure choriocarcinoma of the testis: A potentially curable lesion. *CA* 32:82–84, 1982.
26. Cajal SRY, Pinango L, Barat F, et al. Metastatic pure choriocarcinoma of the testis in an elderly man. *J Urol* 137:516–519, 1987.
27. Scully RE. Testicular tumors with endocrine manifestations. In: *Endocrinology,* vol 3, de Groot LJ, Besser GM, Cahill GF, et al, eds. Philadelphia, WB Saunders Co, 1989, chap 134.
28. Manivel JC, Niehans G, Wick MR, Dehner LP. Intermediate trophoblast in germ cell neoplasms. *Am J Surg Pathol* 11:693–701, 1987.
29. Ulbright TM, Loehrer PJ. Choriocarcinoma-like lesions in patients with testicular germ cell tumors: Two histologic variants. *Am J Surg Pathol* 12:531–541, 1988.
30. Evans RW. Developmental stages of embryo-like bodies in teratoma testis. *J Clin Pathol* 10:31–39, 1957.
31. Parkinson C, Beilby JOW. Features of prognostic significance in testicular germ cell tumors. *J Clin Pathol* 30:113–119, 1977.
32. Friedman NB, Moore RA. Tumors of the testis: A report of 922 cases. *Mil Surg* 99:573–593, 1946.
33. Tapper D, Lack EE. Teratomas in infancy and childhood: A 54-year experience at the Children's Hospital Medical Center. *Ann Surg* 198:398–410, 1983.
34. Ahmed T, Bosl GJ, Hajdu SI. Teratoma with malignant transformation in germ cell tumors in men. *Cancer* 56:860–863, 1985.
35. Berdjis CC, Mostofi FK. Carcinoid tumors of the testis. *J Urol* 118:777–782, 1977.
36. Talerman A, Gratama S, Miranda S. Okagaki T. Primary carcinoid tumor of the testis: Case report, ultrastructure and review of the literature. *Cancer* 42:2696–2706, 1978.

37. Hosking DH, Bowman DM, McMorris SL, Ramsey EW. Primary carcinoid of the testis with metastases. *J Urol* 125:255–256, 1981.

38. Aguirre P, Scully RE. Primitive neuroectodermal tumor of the testis: Report of a case. *Arch Pathol Lab Med* 107:643–645, 1983.

39. Warfel KA, Eble JN, Faught P, Sledge GW, Hull MT. Morphologic spectrum of primitive neural tumors arising in mixed germ cell testicular tumors. *Lab Invest* 60:103A, 1989.

40. Jacobsen GK, Barlebo H, Olsen J, et al. Testicular germ cell tumors in Denmark 1976–1980: Pathology of 1058 consecutive cases. *Acta Radiol Oncol* 23:239–247, 1984.

41. Alderdice JM, Merret JD. Factors influencing the survival of patients with testicular teratoma. *J Clin Pathol* 38:791–796, 1985.

42. Brawn, PN. The origin of germ cell tumors of the testis. *Cancer* 51:1610–1614, 1983.

43. Cardosa de Almeida PC, Scully RE. Diffuse embryoma of the testis: A distinctive form of mixed germ cell tumor. *Am J Surg Pathol* 7:633–642, 1983.

44. Rahlf G, Aeikens B, Truss F, Gregl A. Die klinische bedeutung extratestikular entstehender hodentumoren. *Urologe A* 15:87–90, 1976.

45. Prym P. Spontanheilung eines bosartigen wahrscheinlich chorionepitheliomatosen Gewachses im Hoden. *Virchows Arch A* 265:239–258, 1927.

46. Azzopardi JG, Mostofi FK, Theiss EA. Lesions of testes observed in certain patients with widespread choriocarcinoma and related tumors: The significance and genesis of hematoxylin-staining bodies in the human testis. *Am J Pathol* 38:207–225, 1961.

47. Azzopardi JG, Hoffbrand AV. Retrogression in testicular seminoma with viable metastases. *J Clin Pathol* 18:135–141, 1965.

48. Bar W, Hedinger Chr. Ausgebrannte (okkulte) hodentumoren: Hodenlasionen bei klinisch scheinbar primar extratesticularen malignen Keimzelltumoren. *Virchows Arch A* 377:67–78, 1977.

49. Burt ME, Javadpour N. Germ-cell tumors in patients with apparently normal testes. *Cancer* 47:1911–1915, 1981.

50. Munro AJ, Duncan W, Webb JN. Extragonadal presentations of germ cell tumours. *Br J Urol* 55:547–554, 1983.

51. Powell S, Hendry WF, Peckham MJ. Occult germ-cell testicular tumours. *Br J Urol* 55:440–444, 1983.

52. Daugaard G, Olsen J, van der Maase H, Rorth M, Skakkebaek NE. Carcinoma-in-situ testis in patients with assumed extragonadal germ-cell tumours. *Lancet* 2:528–530, 1987.

53. Azzopardi JG, Hoffbrand AV. Retrogression in testicular seminoma with viable metastases. *J Clin Pathol* 18:135–141, 1965.

54. Oosterhuis JW, Suurmeyer AJH, Sleyfer DTH, Koops HS, Oldhoff J, Fleuren G. Effects of multiple-drug chemotherapy (cis-diammine-dichloroplatinum, bleomycin, and vinblastine) on the maturation of retroperitoneal lymph node

metastases of nonseminomatous germ cell tumors of the testis: No evidence for de novo induction of differentiation. *Cancer* 51:408–416, 1983.

55. McCartney AE, Paradinas FJ, Newlands ES. Significance of the 'maturation' of metastases from germ cell tumors after intensive chemotherapy. *Histopathology* 8:457–467, 1984.
56. Loehrer PJ, Hui S, Clark S, Seal M, et al. Teratoma following cisplatin-based combination chemotherapy for nonseminomatous germ cell tumors: A clinicopathological correlation. *J Urol* 135:1183–1189, 1986.
57. Logothetis CJ, Samuels ML, Trindade A, Johnson DE. The growing teratoma syndrome. *Cancer* 50:1629–1635, 1982.
58. Ulbright TM, Loehrer PJ, Roth LM, Einhorn LH, et al. The development of non-germ cell malignancies within germ cell tumors: A clinicopathologic study of 11 cases. *Cancer* 54:1824–1833, 1984.
59. Ahlgren AD, Simrell CR, Triche TJ, Ozols R, Barsky SH. Sarcoma arising in a residual testicular teratoma after cytoreductive chemotherapy. *Cancer* 54:2015–2018, 1984.
60. Ritchey ML, Bagnall JW, McDonald EC, Sago AL. Development of nongerm cell malignancies in nonseminomatous germ cell tumors. *J Urol* 134:146–149, 1985.

Intratubular Germ Cell Neoplasia 4

The designation "intratubular germ cell neoplasia" refers to the presence of cytologically malignant germ cells within the testicular tubules. The intratubular findings range from the presence of atypical germ cells with cytological and immunocytochemical features of seminoma cells distributed along the basement membranes of the tubules (intratubular germ cell neoplasia, unclassified) to complete replacement of tubules by one or another form of germ cell tumor, such as seminoma or embryonal carcinoma (Table 4.1) (Figures 4.1 to 4.8).

Intratubular Germ Cell Neoplasia, Unclassified

Atypical germ cells have been known to be present in testicular tubules adjacent to both seminomas and nonseminomatous germ cell tumors for many decades.[1] The occurrence of such cells in a testis lacking an invasive tumor and the significance of this phenomenon were not subjects of interest, however, until relatively recently.[2,3] The term "carcinoma in situ" has been used most often to describe the presence of intratubular atypical germ cells, but the designation "intratubular germ cell neoplasia, unclassified" (IGCNU) is more accurate.[4] Carcinoma in situ indicates a process that may progress to invasive carcinoma, but some of the intratubular lesions so designated are followed by the development of a seminoma or a teratoma, neither of which is a carcinoma. Since the intratubular lesion may be followed by the development of a nonseminomatous germ cell tumor as well as a seminoma, the

Table 4.1
Classification of Intratubular Germ Cell Neoplasia

Intratubular germ cell neoplasia, unclassified (carcinoma in situ; intratubular atypical germ cells)
Intratubular germ cell neoplasia, unclassified, with extratubular infiltration
Intratubular seminoma
Typical
Spermatocytic
Intratubular embryonal carcinoma
Intratubular germ cell neoplasia, other forms

atypical germ cells, although indistinguishable from seminoma cells, should be considered totipotent and not intratubular seminoma. The latter term is appropriate only when the tubules are filled with cells having the typical features of seminoma cells (Figure 4.3).[4,5]

IGCNU (Figures 4.1, 4.2), has been seen not only in testicular tissue adjacent to invasive germ cell tumors,[4–9] but in the following other situations as well: (1) in the testes of some patients with extratesticular germ cell tumors and clinically negative testes, as mentioned earlier (page 46)[10–12]; (2) in testicular biopsy specimens from infertile men with small testes and oligospermia[13–18]; (3) in cryptorchid testes both before and after orchidopexy[19–21]; (4) in the testis contralateral to a testis that contains an invasive germ cell tumor or intratubular germ cell neoplasia[22,23]; and (5) in the abnormal testes of patients with intersexual disorders such as mixed gonadal dysgenesis and the androgen insensitivity syndrome (see Chapter 6).

IGCNU is seen in tubules adjacent to invasive germ cell tumors in 75% to 99% of the cases, more frequently in association with nonseminomatous tumors than with seminomas.[4] The lesion has not been described in the tubules of prepubertal patients with yolk sac tumors.[24]

As discussed in the previous chapter, IGCNU is often detected in biopsy or orchidectomy specimens of patients with extratesticular germ cell tumors and clinically uninvolved testes. It was found in 53% of patients with retroperitoneal germ cell tumors with or without mediastinal and visceral metastasis in the series reported by Daugaard et al,[12] but was not observed in cases of mediastinal germ cell neoplasia in the absence of additional retroperitoneal tumor.

In one of the earliest studies of infertile patients with small testes and oligospermia, Skakkebaek[14] found IGCNU in 1.1% of the cases. The changes were bilateral in one third of the positive cases, and in two thirds of them an invasive germ cell tumor was detected within 1.3 to 4.5 years. In a later study of over 2000 infertile men, the lesion was found in eight (0.4%) of the cases.[17] In six of these patients, an invasive germ cell tumor developed during follow-up periods of up to nine years. Although the question arises whether atypical cells in small specimens might be absent as a result of a sampling problem, Berthelsen and Skakkebaek[16] have demonstrated the high probability of detecting the lesion by obtaining two random biopsy specimens 3 mm in diameter.[16]

Krabbe et al[19] examined testicular biopsy specimens from 50 men with a history of cryptorchidism. They found pure IGCNU in two patients and IGCNU accompanied by an invasive germ cell tumor in two other patients. In another series, one third of men with IGCNU had a history of cryptorchidism,[20] and the lesion has also been demonstrated in the cryptorchid testes of four of 117 prepubertal boys.[21]

Since it is well known that patients with a testicular germ cell tumor are at increased risk for a tumor of the contralateral testis, it is not surprising that biopsy specimens of the latter testis in such patients have shown IGCNU in 5% to 8% of the cases.[22,23]

Cumulative follow-up studies indicate that in the majority of the cases patients with IGCNU subsequently have an invasive germ cell tumor of some type, more often a seminoma than a nonseminomatous neoplasm. In some cases, the invasive tumor has not been detected until a decade or more after the diagnosis of the IGCNU.[4]

Microscopic features

In the earliest stage of IGCNU in the postpubertal testis, atypical germ cells appear in small numbers along the basement membranes of tubules that are the site of active spermatogenesis. Later, the spermatogenic epithelium disappears as the atypical germ cells proliferate (Figure 4.1), pushing the remaining Sertoli cells toward the center of the tubule. Concomitant with the proliferation of atypical germ cells, the lamina propria of the tubule typically becomes thickened and hyalinized. The atypical germ cells closely resemble seminoma cells, with abundant clear cytoplasm and nuclei that contain one or a few prominent nucleoli and clumped chromatin (Figure 4.2). Mitotic figures, including atypical forms, may be present. The cytoplasm contains large amounts of glycogen (Figure 4.4) in contrast to spermatogonia, which contain relatively little. The cytoplasm of the atypical cells stained immunohistochemically for ferritin in 82% of the cases in one study,[25] but another group found such staining in only 2% to 3% of cases.[7] Staining for placental-like alkaline phosphatase is positive in 80% to 100% of cases[26,27]; the cells also can be stained for neuron-specific enolase.

When IGCNU is seen in the prepubertal testis, as in cases of cryptorchidism, the androgen insensitivity syndrome, and mixed gonadal dysgenesis, the involved tubules resemble those of the normal prepubertal testis except for the presence of the atypical germ cells.[28]

The cells of IGCNU may break through the lamina propria of the tubules and invade the stroma in small clusters (Figures 4.9, 4.10), or they may continue to proliferate and fill the tubules, forming an intratubular seminoma (Figure 4.3). The invasive lesion has been referred to both as IGCNU with extratubular infiltration and as microinvasive germ cell tumor.[29] Like the intratubular lesion, the microinvasive lesion may be followed by the development of either a seminoma or a nonseminomatous germ cell tumor.

The management of patients with IGCNU remains controversial. Regular testicular self-examination with frequent follow-up examinations by the physician, using various techniques for early detection of testicular cancer, is one approach; orchidectomy is another. Chemotherapy eradicates the lesion in some, but not all cases; low-dose radiation therapy has been shown to destroy the lesion.[30]

Intratubular Seminoma

Intratubular seminoma is less common than IGCNU and, in contrast, has a higher frequency of association with seminomas (44%) than with nonseminomatous germ cell tumors (27%).[4] Intratubular seminoma with syncytiotrophoblast cells has been encountered rarely. Intratubular spermatocytic seminoma is often present within tubules outside an invasive spermatocytic seminoma, often at a distance from it; we have seen one example of entirely intratubular spermatocytic seminoma (Figures 4.7, 4.8).

Intratubular Embryonal Carcinoma

Intratubular embryonal carcinoma is characterized by distension of tubules by solid plugs of cells resembling those of invasive embryonal carcinoma. Extensive caseationlike necrosis is often present (Figure 4.5), with basophilic deposits frequently observed in the center of the intraluminal necrotic material (Figure 4.6). The lesion has been observed adjacent to nonseminomatous germ cell tumors and in clinically negative testes in patients with an extratesticular presentation of a nonseminomatous germ cell tumor. Isolated syncytiotrophoblast cells have also been identified within tubules.

Other Forms of Intratubular Germ Cell Neoplasia

In rare cases of yolk sac tumor in children, intratubular yolk sac tumor has been observed adjacent to the invasive tumor.[31] Intratubular teratoma has not been described in humans.

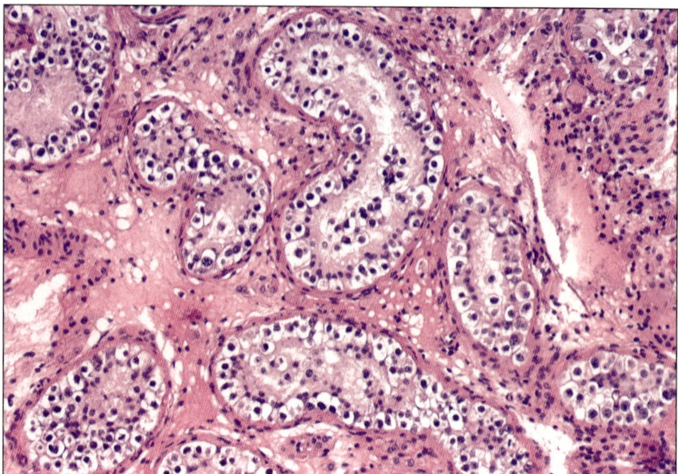

Figure 4.1 Intratubular germ cell neoplasia, unclassified. All of the tubules contain along their basement membranes large cells with clear cytoplasm and central nuclei resembling the cells of seminoma. The normal spermatogenic epithelium has disappeared, but occasional Sertoli cells can be seen.

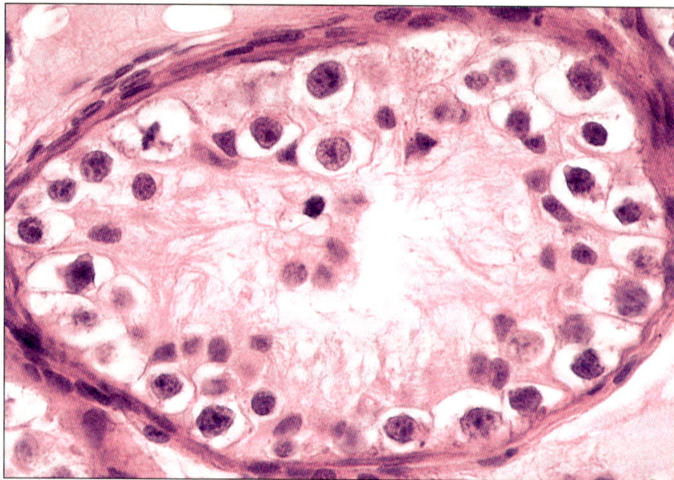

Figure 4.2 Intratubular germ cell neoplasia, unclassified. The tumor cells have the appearance of seminoma cells with clear cytoplasm and rounded nuclei containing prominent nucleoli. One mitotic figure is visible. Occasional Sertoli cells with small nuclei are also present.

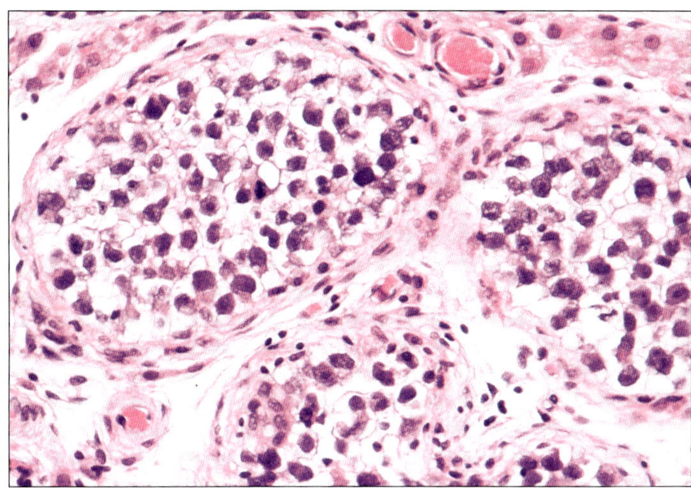

Figure 4.3 Intratubular seminoma. Cells resembling seminoma cells fill the tubules.

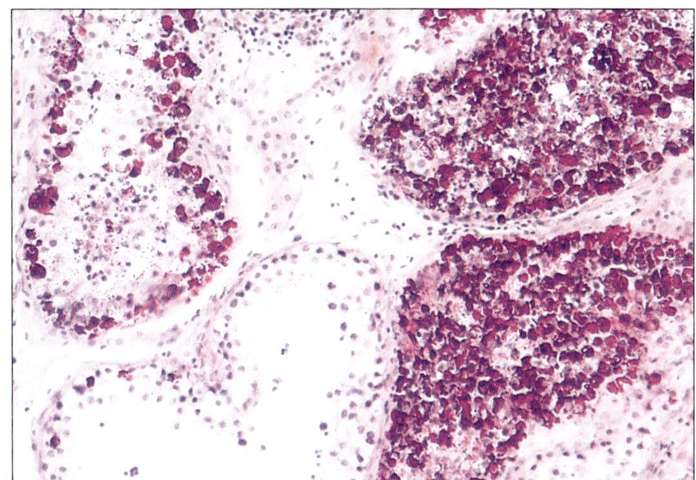

Figure 4.4 Intratubular seminoma (right) and intratubular germ cell neoplasia, unclassified (left). The neoplastic cells are stained for glycogen by the PAS technique.

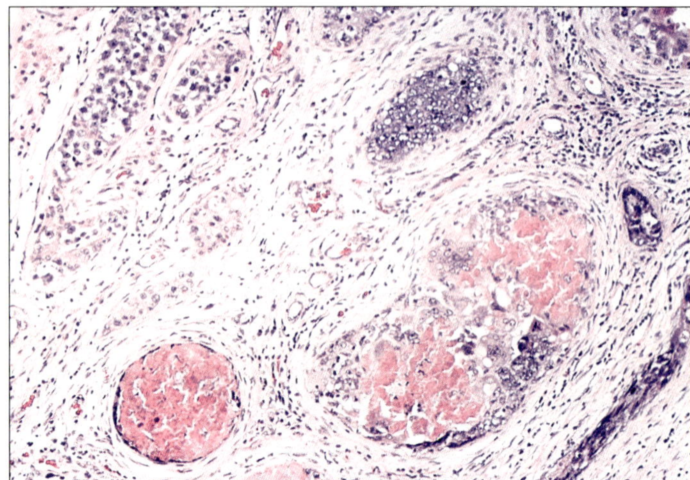

Figure 4.5 Intratubular embryonal carcinoma and intratubular seminoma. The intratubular embryonal carcinoma is characterized by larger, darker cells than the intratubular seminoma and is necrotic in several of the tubules.

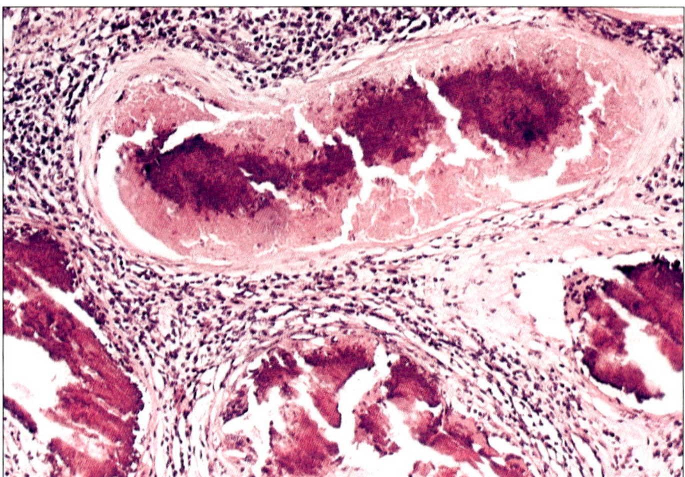

Figure 4.6 Intratubular embryonal carcinoma. The intratubular tumor has undergone complete necrosis with the central deposition of basophilic material.

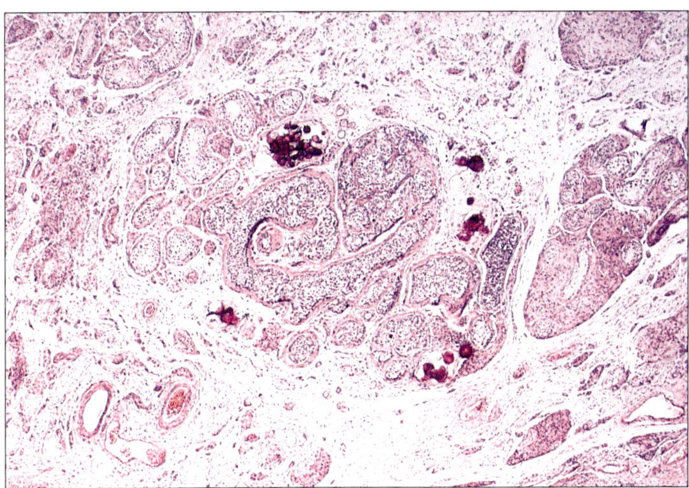

Figure 4.7 Intratubular spermatocytic seminoma. Centrally located tubules are filled with spermatocytic seminoma cells. Several tubules have calcified contents.

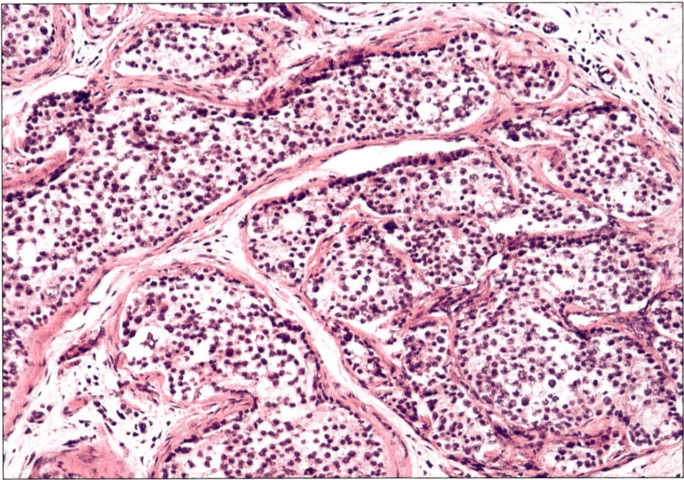

Figure 4.8 Intratubular spermatocytic seminoma. The tubules are filled with cells containing round nuclei of varying sizes.

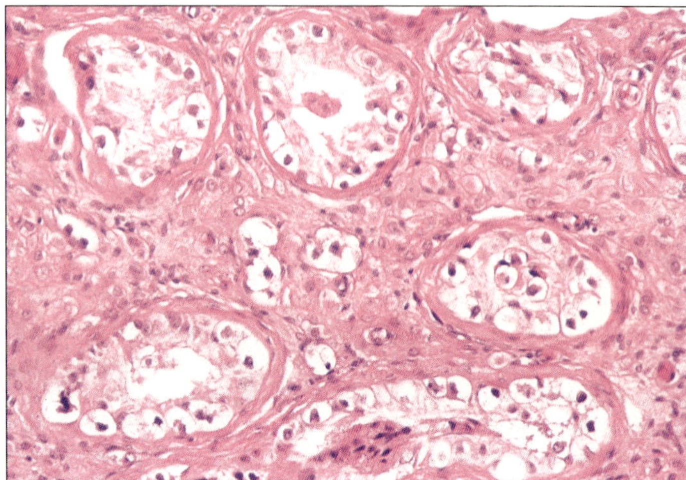

Figure 4.9 Intratubular germ cell neoplasia, unclassified with extratubular infiltration. Small clusters of cells resembling seminoma cells are present in the stroma. Intratubular tumor cells are also seen.

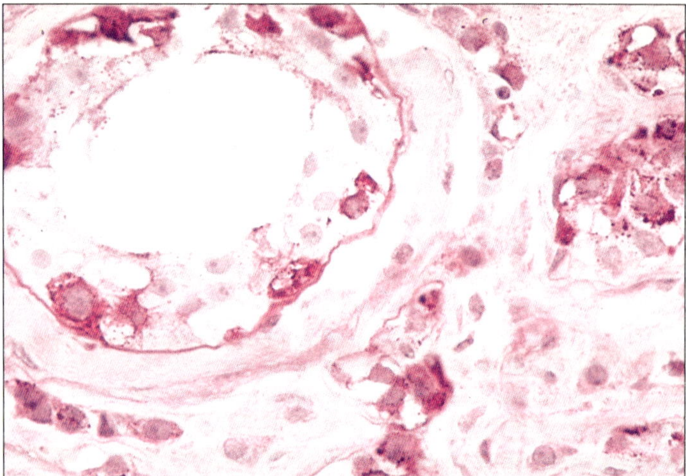

Figure 4.10 Intratubular germ cell neoplasia, unclassified with extratubular infiltration. Both the intratubular and the extratubular tumor are stained for glycogen by the PAS technique. The basement membrane of the tubule is also stained.

References

1. Mark EJ, Hedinger C. Changes in remaining tumor-free testicular tissue in cases of seminoma and teratoma. *Virchows Arch A* 340:84–92, 1965.
2. Skakkebaek NE. Abnormal morphology of germ cells in two infertile men. *Acta Pathol Microbiol Scand A* 80:374–378, 1972.
3. Skakkebaek NE. Possible carcinoma-in-situ of the testis. *Lancet* 2:516–517, 1972.
4. Scully RE. Testis. In: *The Pathology of Incipient Neoplasia,* Henson DE, Albores-Saavedra J, eds. Philadelphia, W.B. Saunders Co, 1986, chap 18.
5. Skakkebaek NE, ed. Carcinoma-in-situ and cancer of the testis. *Int J Androl* 10:1–430, 1987.
6. Skakkebaek NE. Atypical germ cells in the adjacent 'normal' tissue of testicular tumors. *Acta Path Microbiol Scand A* 83:127–130, 1975.
7. Jacobsen GK, Henriksen OB, Der Maase HV. Carcinoma in situ of testicular tissue adjacent to malignant germ-cell tumors: A study of 105 cases. *Cancer* 47:2660–2662, 1981.
8. Klein FA, Melamed MR, Whitmore WF Jr. Intratubular malignant germ cells (carcinoma in situ) accompanying invasive testicular germ cell tumors. *J Urol* 133:413–415, 1985.
9. Coffin CM, Ewing S, Dehner LP. Frequency of intratubular germ cell neoplasia with invasive testicular germ cell tumors: Histologic and immunocytochemical features. *Arch Pathol Lab Med* 109:555–559, 1985.
10. Azzopardi JG, Mostofi FK, Theiss EA. Lesions of testes observed in certain patients with widespread choriocarcinoma and related tumors: The significance and genesis of hematoxylin-staining bodies in the human testis. *Am J Pathol* 38:207–255, 1961.
11. Richter HJ, Leder L–D. Lymph node metastases with PAS-positive tumor cells and massive epithelioid granulomatous reaction as diagnostic clues to occult seminoma. *Cancer* 44:245–249, 1979.
12. Daugaard G, Von der Maase H, Olsen J, Rorth M, Skakkebaek NE. Carcinoma-in-situ testis in patients with assumed extragonadal germ-cell tumours. *Lancet* 2:528–529, 1987.
13. Skakkebaek NE, Berthelsen JG. Carcinoma-in-situ of testis and orchiectomy. *Lancet* 2:204–205, 1978.
14. Skakkebaek NE. Carcinoma in situ of the testis: Frequency and relationship to invasive germ cell tumours in infertile men. *Histopathology* 2:157–170, 1978.
15. Andres TL, Trainer TD, Leadbetter GW. Atypical germ cells preceding metachronous bilateral testicular tumors. *Urology* 15:307–309, 1980.
16. Berthelsen JG, Skakkebaek NE. Value of testicular biopsy in diagnosing carcinoma in situ testis. *Scand J Urol Nephrol* 15:165–168, 1981.
17. Pryor JP, Cameron KM, Chilton CP, et al. Carcinoma in situ in testicular biopsies from men presenting with infertility. *Br J Urol* 55:780–784, 1983.

18. West AB, Butler MR, Fitzpatrick J, O'Brien A. Testicular tumors in subfertile men: Report of 4 cases with implications for management of patients presenting with infertility. *J Urol* 133:107–109, 1985.

19. Krabbe S, Berthelsen JG, Volsted P, et al: High incidence of undetected neoplasia in maldescended testes. *Lancet* 1:999–1000, 1979.

20. Skakkebaek, NE, Berthelsen JG, Muller J. Carcinoma-in-situ of the undescended testis. *Urol Clin North Am* 9:377–385, 1982.

21. Aneiros J, Zuluaga A, Lopez J, et al. Atypical germ cells in prepubertal cryptorchid testes. *Br J Urol* 60:258–260, 1987.

22. Berthelsen JG, Skakkebaek NE, Mogensen P, Sorensen BL. Incidence of carcinoma in situ of germ cells in contralateral testes of men with testicular tumors. *Br Med J* 2:363–364, 1979.

23. Von der Masse H, Rorth M, Walbom-Jorgensen S, et al: Carcinoma-in-situ of contralateral testis in patients with testicular germ cell cancer: Study of 27 cases in 500 patients. *Br Med J* 293:1398–1401, 1986.

24. Manivel JC, Simonton S, Wold LE, Dehner LP: Absence of intratubular germ cell neoplasia in testicular yolk sac tumors in children: A histochemical and immunohistochemical study. *Arch Pathol Lab Med* 112:641–645, 1988.

25. Jacobsen GK, Jacobsen M, Clausen PP: Ferritin as a possible marker protein of carcinoma-in-situ of the testis. *Lancet* 2:533–534, 1970.

26. Jacobsen GK, Norgaard-Pedersen B: Placental alkaline phosphatase in testicular germ cell tumours and in carcinoma-in-situ of the testis. *Acta Pathol Microbiol Immunol Scand A* 92:323–329, 1984.

27. Burke AP, Mostofi FK. Intratubular malignant germ cells in testicular biopsies: Clinical course and identification by staining for placental alkaline phosphatase. *Mod Pathol* 1:475–479, 1988.

28. Muller J: *Abnormal Infantile Germ Cells and Development of Carcinoma-in-Situ in Maldeveloped Testes*. Boston, Blackwell Scientific Publications, 1987, p 26.

29. Von Eyben FE, Mikulowski P, Busch C: Microinvasive germ cell tumors of the testis. *J Urol* 126:842–844, 1981.

30. Von der Maase H, Giwercman A, Muller J, Skakkebaek NE. Management of carcinoma-in-situ. *Int J Androl* 10:209–220, 1987.

31. Mostofi FK. Pathology of germ cell tumors of the testis: A progress report. *Cancer* 45:1735–1754, 1980.

Sex Cord–Stromal Tumors 5

Included in this category are neoplasms that contain cells resembling Sertoli cells, Leydig cells, granulosa cells, and theca cells, as well as fibroblasts in varying combinations and varying degrees of differentiation.[1,2] These tumors account for approximately 4% of testicular neoplasms. Most of the reported cases have been Leydig cell tumors; smaller numbers of Sertoli cell tumors and rare granulosa cell tumors have also been described. The remaining neoplasms in this category have contained cells of both testicular and ovarian types or cells that cannot be specifically identified as either.[1] With the exception of Leydig cell tumors, sex cord–stromal tumors of the testis are encountered unusually frequently in prepubertal children, in whom over one third of them occur.

Leydig Cell Tumors

Leydig cell tumors account for 1% to 3% of testicular neoplasms.[3] They occur at all ages, but are most common between 20 and 50 years of age. Adult patients usually complain of testicular swelling, but gynecomastia is the initial symptom in 15% of them. Children with a Leydig cell tumor almost invariably present with isosexual pseudoprecocity, which typically appears between the ages of 5 and 9 years.

Approximately 3% of Leydig cell tumors are bilateral and the tumor has extended beyond the testis at the time of presentation in 10% to 15% of the cases.[3] The tumors are typically sharply circumscribed (Figures 5.1, 5.2), are usually 3 to 5 cm in diameter, and are sometimes lobulated by fibrous septa (Figure 5.2). The neoplastic tissue is almost always uniformly solid and usually yellow (Figure 5.1) or yellow-tan, but occasionally it is gray-white, brown (Figure 5.3), or green-brown (Figure 5.2). Foci of hemorrhage, necrosis (Figure 5.3), or both are present in 25% of the cases.[3]

The most common microscopic pattern is diffuse (Figure 5.4), although insular, trabecular (Figure 5.5), pseudotubular, and ribbonlike arrangements of the tumor cells are also encountered (Figure 5.6). The stroma is typically inconspicuous, but occasionally it is prominent; it may be hyalinized and it sometimes forms broad bands intersecting the tumor tissue. Less commonly, the stroma is edematous or myxoid; rarely, a stroma with these features is conspicuous (Figure 5.6).

The neoplastic cells are typically large and polygonal with abundant eosinophilic, slightly granular cytoplasm (Figure 5.7); occasionally the cytoplasm is extensively vacuolated or spongy as a result of lipid accumulation (Figure 5.8). Rarely, the cells are spindle-shaped (Figure 5.9) or are small with scanty cytoplasm and have nuclei containing grooves. Crystals of Reinke (Figure 5.10) have been identified in the cytoplasm in approximately one third of the cases and lipochrome pigment has been found in 10% to 15%.[3] In one reported case,[4] occasional psammoma bodies were scattered within the tumor (Figure 5.11). The nuclei are typically round and contain a single prominent nucleolus. Nuclear atypicality is usually absent or of a minor degree, but is marked in some tumors (Figure 5.12). The mitotic rate varies greatly. It is usually low, but is high in occasional tumors (Figures 5.9, 5.13).

No single pathologic criterion reliably distinguishes a benign from a malignant Leydig cell tumor. However, the latter are typically larger than the former, have infiltrative margins, invade lymphatics or blood vessels, and contain foci of necrosis. They also have a high mitotic rate (more than three per ten high-power fields) and significant nuclear atypicality much more often than tumors that have a benign outcome. When a number of the above features are present, the possibility of a clinically malignant course is significantly increased. All five tumors that were clinically malignant in the series of 40 tumors reported by Kim et al[3] had four or more of the above features. In contrast, 12 of the 14 tumors that appeared to be benign on the basis of follow-up data of two or more years' duration had none of these features. One benign tumor had only one such feature and one had three such features.

Leydig cell tumors may be confused with malignant lymphomas or plasmacytomas, particularly when their cells contain less than the usual amount of cytoplasm and have atypical nuclei. Features of lymphomas that are helpful in the differential diagnosis include a much higher frequency of bilaterality (up to 38%), the common presence of invasion of the epididymis and spermatic cord, characteristic intertubular infiltration of the tumor cells, invasion of the tubules in one third of the cases, and the distinctive cytologic features of the neoplastic cells. Metastatic carcinoma, particularly of prostatic origin, is occasionally mistaken for a Leydig cell tumor when the former has a diffuse pattern. In such cases the clinical history and the presence of other areas characteristic of prostatic adenocarcinoma are helpful diagnostically; immunocytochemical staining for prostate-specific acid phosphatase and prostate-specific antigen is almost always diagnostic. Leydig cell tumors are generally relatively easily distinguished from other tumors in the sex cord–stromal category because the resemblance of the neoplastic cells to Leydig cells is usually sufficiently striking to suggest the correct diagnosis. Occasionally, however, the rare Leydig cell tumor that contains cells with nuclear grooves may focally resemble a granulosa cell tumor and a pseudotubular or trabecular pattern in a Leydig cell tumor may suggest the diagnosis of a Sertoli cell tumor. Tumors with such confusing features, however, usually have foci of typical Leydig cell neoplasia elsewhere within the specimen. The differentiation of Leydig cell tumors from large cell calcifying Sertoli cell tumors and from the tumorlike masses that develop in the testes of patients with the adrenogenital syndrome are discussed on pages 106 and 190, respectively.

Malakoplakia may also be confused with a Leydig cell tumor because it typically results in the formation of a homogenous, yellow or brown mass. The gross finding of an abscess, which is present in most cases of malakoplakia, is an important clue to the diagnosis. On low-power microscopic examination the diagnosis of a Leydig cell tumor is also often suggested because the testicular parenchyma is replaced by large cells with abundant granular eosinophilic cytoplasm (von Hansemann cells). These cells, however, occupy tubules as well as the interstitium and are typically admixed with other inflammatory cells. In addition, many of the cells contain in their cytoplasm round to oval, basophilic inclusions (Michaelis-Gutmann bodies).

The majority of patients with a Leydig cell tumor have a good prognosis. In the largest series of these tumors reported to date, metastatic disease developed in five of the 30 patients on whom follow-up data were obtained.[3] One additional patient in that series had a Leydig cell tumor of the contralateral testis 16 years after excision of the initial tumor; he was well four years after the second operation. As noted above, a number of features viewed in aggregate are helpful in assessing the likelihood of a malignant course in a given case. The primary treatment of a Leydig cell tumor is inguinal orchiectomy. If the gross or histologic features suggest that a clinically malignant behavior is likely, the performance of a retroperitoneal lymphadenectomy should be considered. The treatment of metastatic Leydig cell tumors by chemotherapy has not proven very satisfactory at the present time.

Sertoli Cell Tumors

General features

The resemblance of some testicular tumors to estrogenic lipid-rich Sertoli cell tumors of the canine testis[5] led to their recognition by Teilum[6,7] as Sertoli cell tumors. Sertoli cell tumors of all types are uncommon, accounting for less than 1% of testicular neoplasms. They occur at all ages, with approximately 15% of the reported cases in children. Four of them have been reported in boys with the Peutz-Jeghers syndrome.[8–11] Such an occurrence is noteworthy because of the frequency of ovarian sex cord tumors with annular tubules, which contain Sertoli cells, in female patients with this syndrome.[12] Also of interest is the focal resemblance of two of the four testicular Sertoli cell tumors associated with the Peutz-Jeghers syndrome[9,11] to the large cell calcifying Sertoli cell tumor of the testis, which has highly distinctive clinical and pathological features, and is discussed separately below. Another distinctive-appearing Sertoli cell tumor, which occurs in the testes of patients with the androgen insensitivity syndrome, is considered in the next chapter.

On gross examination, Sertoli cell tumors are typically well circumscribed, sometimes lobulated, yellow, tan or white masses; occasionally foci of hemorrhage are present (Figure 5.14). Microscopic examination reveals tubules that are sometimes hollow (Figure 5.15), but are usually solid (Figure 5.16), and cords, nests, and masses of cells (Figure 5.17) compatible with Sertoli cells. The tumor cells may contain abundant intracytoplasmic lipid, usually as fine droplets, but occasionally in large vacuoles (Figure 5.18) resembling those of the estrogenic canine Sertoli cell tumor.[4] The stroma may be scanty or composed of abundant fibrous tissue that may be hyalinized (Figure 5.19). Most Sertoli cell tumors are well differentiated and benign, but occasional examples are less well differentiated and pursue a malignant course (Figures 5.20, 5.21). It is impossible to determine the frequency of malignancy of Sertoli cell tumors because of limited follow-up data in most of the reported cases and the difficulty distinguishing pure Sertoli cell tumors from sex cord–stromal tumors with a Sertoli cell component on the basis of published reports in the literature.

Sertoli cell tumors must be distinguished from focal nonneoplastic clusters of small tubules (Figure 5.22) that are lined by immature Sertoli cells and, in occasional cases, contain scattered spermatogonia as well. In some lesions, small hyaline bodies resembling Call-Exner bodies or laminated calcified bodies are found within the tubules (Figure 5.23). These lesions are usually microscopic, but are occasionally visible grossly as white nodules a few millimeters in diameter. Although encountered much more often in cryptorchid than in scrotal testes, they have been found in up to 22% of the latter.[13] They have sometimes been referred to as tubular adenomas or Sertoli cell adenomas, but are presently regarded as hyperplastic nodules of immature cells rather than neoplasms.

Because of their typically prominent tubular differentiation, the distinction of pure Sertoli cell tumors from other sex cord–stromal tumors, and indeed, from other testicular tumors in general, is rarely difficult. In occasional tumors, however, a tubular pattern may be inconspicuous in part of the specimen and other diagnoses may be considered. For example, some Sertoli cell tumors have a diffuse pattern (Figure 5.17) that may simulate the pattern of a Leydig cell tumor. Conversely, other tumors such as metastatic carcinoma and rare seminomas may have a tubular pattern. Such tumors should be excluded before a diagnosis of Sertoli cell tumor is made.

Large cell calcifying Sertoli cell tumor

This recently recognized subtype of Sertoli cell tumor has a variety of unusual clinical and pathologic features.[14] The ages of the patients have ranged from five to 44 years, with an average of 16 years. In almost half the reported cases a variety of associated lesions, including pituitary adenomas, bilateral primary adrenocortical hyperplasia, testicular Leydig cell tumors, cardiac myxomas, and spotty mucocutaneous pigmentation have been present.[15] Clinical associations have included acromegaly, pituitary gigantism, hypercortisolemia, sexual precocity, sudden death, and the Peutz-Jeghers syndrome.

The tumors are usually 4 cm or less in diameter, although in one case a large tumor replaced the entire testis; they are often multifocal and are bilateral in approximately 40% of the cases. Sectioning discloses firm, yellow (Figure 5.24) to tan tissue in which granular calcific foci may be detectable; the tumors appear grossly well circumscribed although microscopic examination reveals ill-defined margins in most of the cases. The neoplastic cells are arranged in diffuse sheets, nests, trabeculae, cords, small clusters, or solid tubules (Figures 5.25 to 5.28). The stroma varies from loose and myxoid (Figure 5.26) to densely collagenous (Figure 5.27). Foci of intratubular tumor are found in approximately one half of the cases (Figure 5.29). A characteristic feature is the presence of calcification, which is usually conspicuous (Figure 5.25) and sometimes massive, with the formation of large, wavy, laminated nodules (Figure 5.30). In rare cases, Sertoli cell tumors have an appearance identical to that of the large cell calcifying Sertoli cell tumor, but lack calcification in the areas that have been sampled (Figures 5.31, 5.32). The neoplastic cells are large and usually rounded, but occasionally are cuboidal or columnar, and rarely are spindle-shaped. In most of the cases, the cytoplasm is abundant, eosinophilic, and finely granular (Figure 5.28), but occasionally it is amphophilic and slightly vacuolated. The nuclei are round or oval with one or two small nucleoli. Mitotic figures are generally rare. Only one tumor, occurring in a 44-year-old man, was microscopically atypical with abnormal nuclear features and aggressive invasion; it was also clinically malignant. Ultrastructural studies support the Sertoli cell origin of the tumor, with the identification of Charcot-Böttcher filament bundles, considered to be specific cytoplasmic inclusions of Sertoli cells, in two cases.[16,17]

The large cell calcifying Sertoli cell tumor may be misinterpreted as a Leydig cell tumor because its cells contain abundant eosinophilic cytoplasm. However, its common multifocality and bilaterality and the presence of intratubular growth and calcification are all either rare or undescribed in Leydig cell tumors. In addition, crystals of Reinke, which are characteristic of Leydig cell tumors, have not been identified in the cells of the large cell calcifying Sertoli cell tumor. Finally, with the exception of a shared association with sexual precocity, the clinical features of both tumors differ greatly.

Granulosa Cell Tumors

Adult type

Granulosa cell tumors of the histologic types encountered in the ovaries of adult women are very rare in the testis.[1,2,18,19] Four of the nine reported cases of such tumors have been associated with gynecomastia.

They have ranged in diameter from 1.8 to 13 cm and have typically been homogeneous, yellow to yellow-gray, firm, and lobulated (Figure 5.33). The microscopic patterns have been mainly microfollicular, with Call-Exner bodies (Figure 5.34), and diffuse (Figure 5.35). The cytoplasm is typically scanty and the nuclei are pale and may have grooves. In some cases, however, the nuclei are larger, rounder, and more hyperchromatic. One adult granulosa cell tumor has been reported to pursue a malignant course.[1]

Because of the characteristic architectural and cytologic features of the adult form of granulosa cell tumor, it should not readily be confused with other tumors. Unclassified tumors in the sex cord–stromal category may have a focal appearance compatible with the diagnosis of a granulosa cell tumor and the specific diagnosis of granulosa cell tumor should only be made when all or almost all the neoplasm has granulosa cell features. As mentioned on page 102, it should be emphasized that rare Leydig cell tumors also contain cells with nuclear grooves.

Juvenile type

Granulosa cell tumors similar to the juvenile granulosa cell tumor of the ovary are the most common neoplasms of the neonatal testis.[20,21] They are usually discovered in the first four months of life, but one of them was first detected in a 21-month-old child.[2] Three cases of testicular juvenile granulosa cell tumor have also been reported in undescended testes of infants with intersexual disorders.[22,23]

The tumors have ranged up to 6 cm in diameter. They may be solid, cystic, or both (Figures 5.36, 5.37); the cysts are thin-walled and contain viscid or gelatinous fluid or clotted blood. Microscopic examination reveals follicular or solid patterns or both (Figure 5.38). The follicles are most often large and round to oval, but may be irregular (Figure 5.39) and typically contain fluid, which may be basophilic (Figure 5.38) or eosinophilic, and is stained by mucicarmine (Figure 5.40). In tumors with a solid pattern, the cells grow in sheets, nodules, and irregular clusters. Hyalinization is often extensive, and in some cases intercellular basophilic mucinous fluid is conspicuous. The tumor cells have moderate to large amounts of pale to eosinophilic cytoplasm (Figure 5.41) and hyperchromatic, round to oval nuclei, some of which contain nucleoli. Mitotic activity may be prominent (Figure 5.42). No juvenile granulosa cell tumor of the testis has been reported to pursue a malignant course.

The juvenile granulosa cell tumor may be misinterpreted as a yolk sac tumor, particularly when it exhibits significant nuclear atypicality and mitotic activity, and the cytoplasm of the tumor cells is pale. The presence of follicles in most juvenile granulosa cell tumors, the absence of various characteristic patterns of yolk sac tumor, and the lack of immunohistochemical staining for AFP should help avoid this misdiagnosis.

Sex Cord–Stromal Tumors, Unclassified

Testicular tumors in the sex cord–stromal category are more difficult to classify within the specific subtypes discussed above than their ovarian counterparts because much more often they lack specific differentiation, or contain cells resembling to varying degrees both testicular and ovarian elements. Tumors with the typical morphologic features of ovarian Sertoli-Leydig cell tumors, granulosa cell tumors, and thecal cell tumors are exceptional, and, therefore, in the testis a much greater proportion of sex cord–stromal tumors are designated as unclassified than in the ovary.

Unclassified sex cord–stromal tumors occur at all ages.[1] The most common clinical symptom is painless testicular enlargement, although gynecomastia is occasionally present. On gross examination the tumors vary greatly in size, with many of them replacing most or all of the testis. They are usually well circumscribed and are composed of white to yellow, often lobulated tissue (Figure 5.43), sometimes traversed by gray-white fibrous septa. Cysts are present in some cases; hemorrhage and necrosis are uncommon.

Microscopic examination reveals a spectrum of patterns, ranging from predominantly epithelial to predominantly stromal (Figures 5.44 to 5.48). The better differentiated tumors typically contain well-formed solid or hollow tubules, or cords (Figure 5.45) composed of or lined by cells resembling Sertoli cells. These cells may be columnar or polyhedral; the cytoplasm varies from scanty to abundant and may be eosinophilic, amphophilic, or vacuolated and lipid-laden; the nuclei are round to oval and often vesicular, and sometimes contain single small nucleoli; mitotic figures are generally rare or absent. Islands and masses of cells resembling granulosa cells (Figure 5.44) and containing Call-Exner–like bodies may also be present (Figure 5.46), but usually the neoplastic cell nuclei lack the features of those of ovarian granulosa cell tumors such as nuclear grooves. The stromal component of the tumors may be densely cellular or fibromatous (Figure 5.47). The less well differentiated tumors exhibit varying degrees of nuclear pleomorphism and mitotic activity. Diffuse and sarcomatoid patterns are frequent, and in some areas it may be difficult or impossible to distinguish the epithelial and stromal components on routine staining. Reticulum stains may help to delineate the two components (Figure 5.48).

As mentioned earlier, the distinction among Sertoli cell tumors, granulosa cell tumors, and unclassified sex cord–stromal tumors is difficult or impossible in many of the cases, including malignant ones, that have been reported in the literature. Among malignant cases in all three categories, only two occurred before puberty,[24,25] while 17 were reported in older patients,[2,26–28] despite the relatively greater frequency of these tumors in children. Indeed, more than one third of the reported tumors in patients over the age of 10 years with follow-up data of one or more years' duration pursued a malignant course.[2] The frequency of distant metastasis appears to be strikingly higher than it is in cases of ovarian sex cord–stromal tumors.[29]

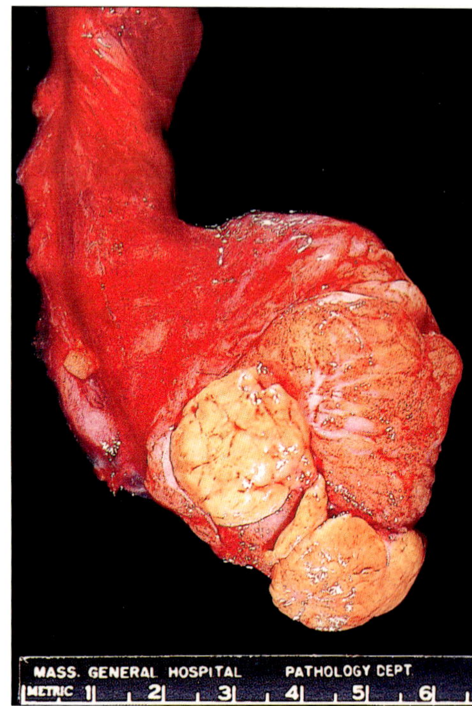

Figure 5.1 Leydig cell tumor. The tumor is well demarcated and yellow.

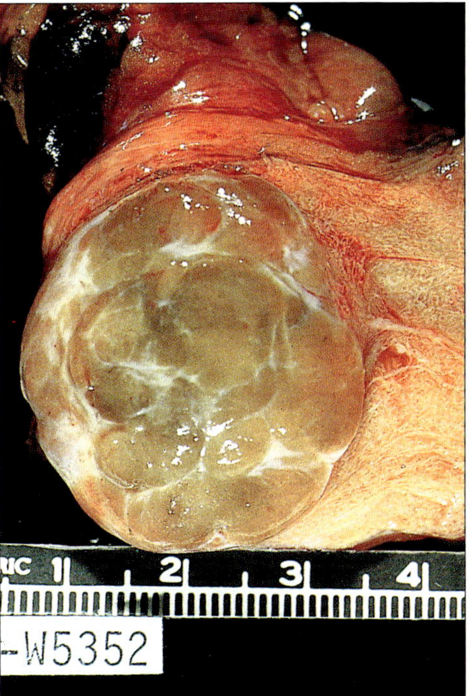

Figure 5.2 Leydig cell tumor. The well-demarcated tumor is pale, brownish-green and lobulated by fibrous tissue septa.

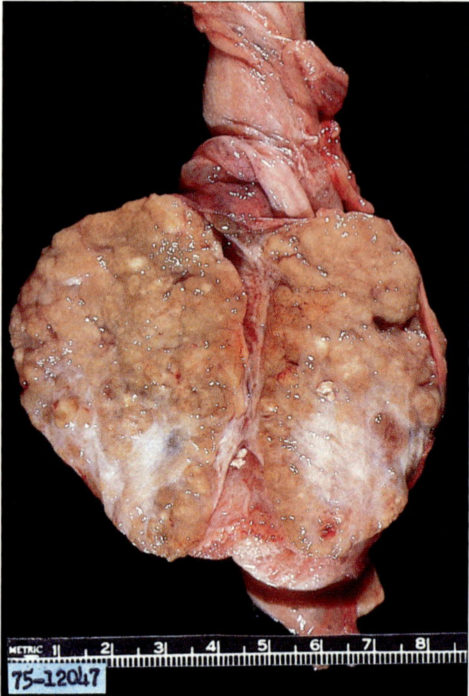

Figure 5.3 Leydig cell tumor. This tumor, which metastasized, is brown and is characterized by lobulation, focal scarring, and a few small yellow foci of necrosis.

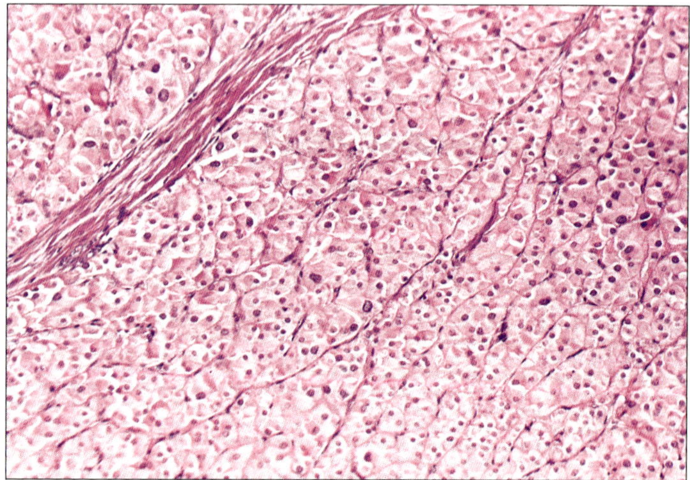

Figure 5.4 Leydig cell tumor. The neoplastic cells have a diffuse pattern with closely packed aggregates separated by numerous thin-walled vessels.

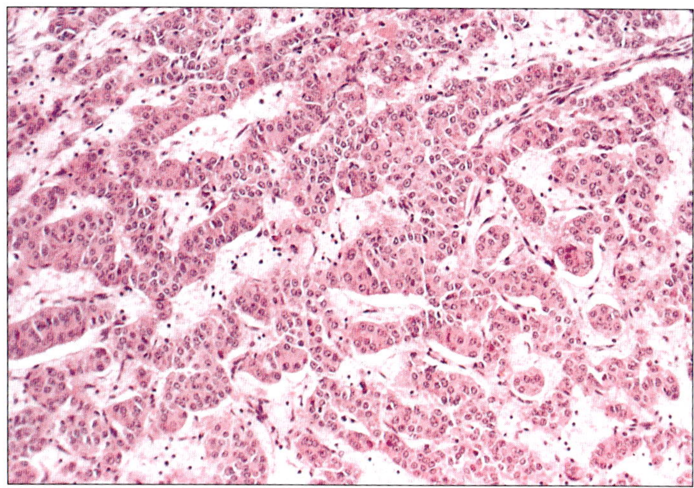

Figure 5.5 Leydig cell tumor. The neoplastic cells are arranged in anastomosing trabeculae.

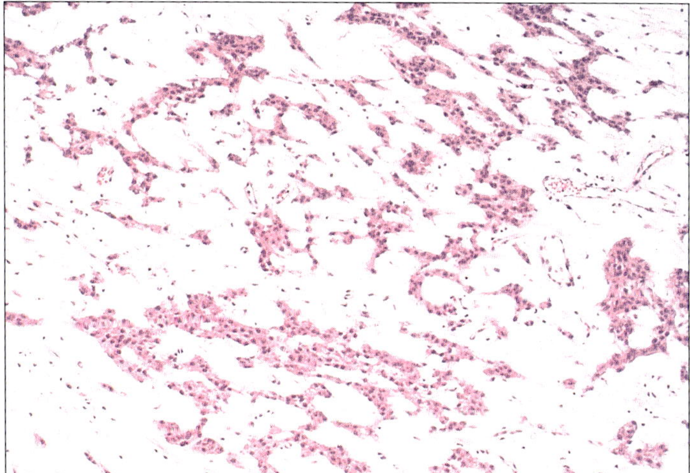

Figure 5.6 Leydig cell tumor. The neoplastic cells are arranged in irregular cords and strands separated by edematous stroma.

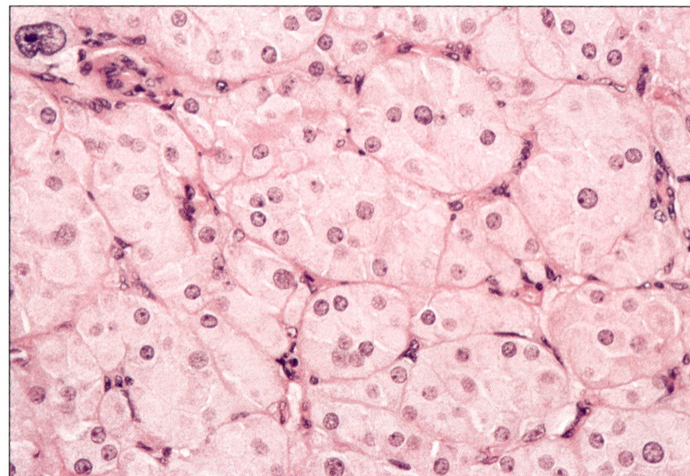

Figure 5.7 Leydig cell tumor. The neoplastic cells contain abundant, finely granular, eosinophilic cytoplasm and central, round nuclei with prominent nucleoli.

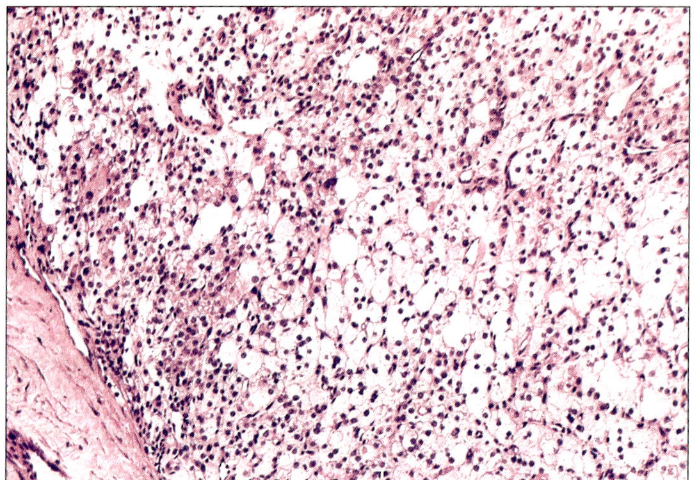

Figure 5.8 Leydig cell tumor. Most of the neoplastic cells are distended by fine, fat vacuoles.

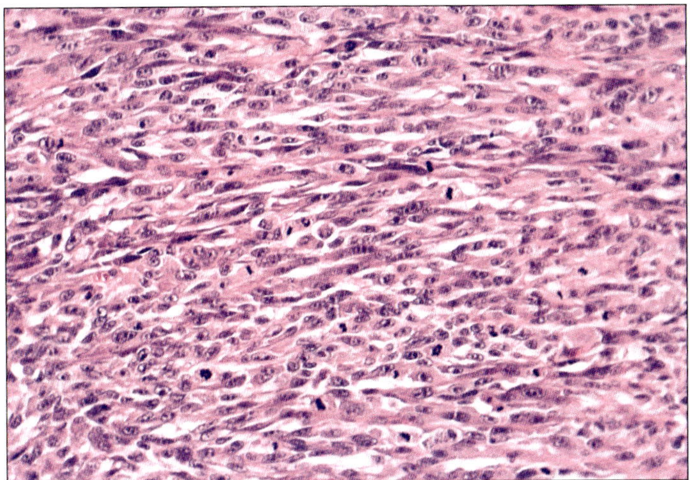

Figure 5.9 Leydig cell tumor. The cells are spindle shaped and have atypical nuclei with numerous mitotic figures.

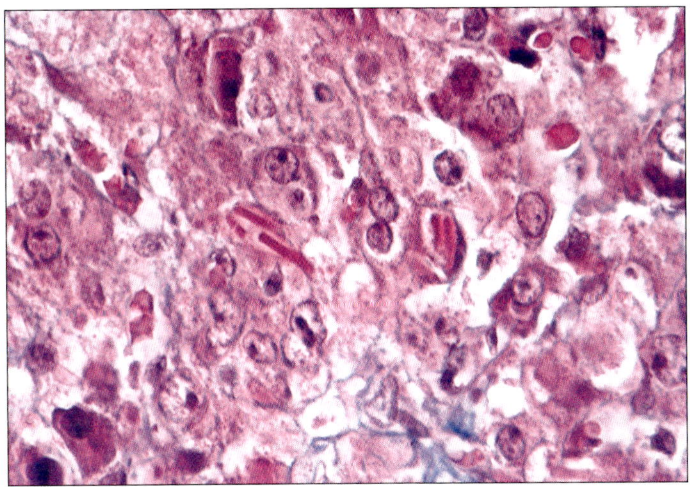

Figure 5.10 Leydig cell tumor. Several crystals of Reinke are stained red by the Masson trichrome technique.

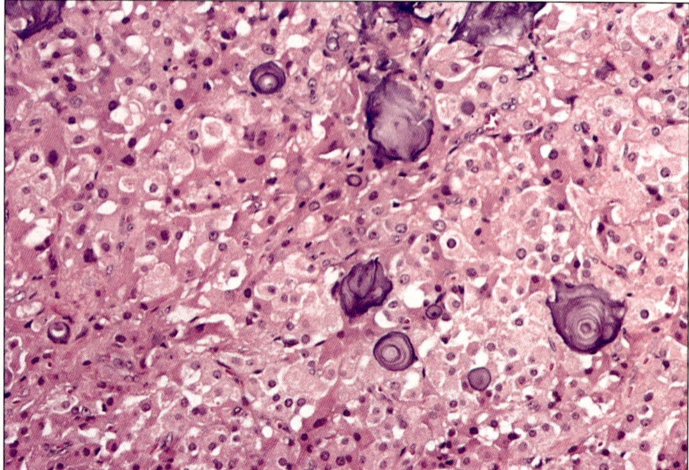

Figure 5.11 Leydig cell tumor. Numerous laminated psammoma bodies are present.

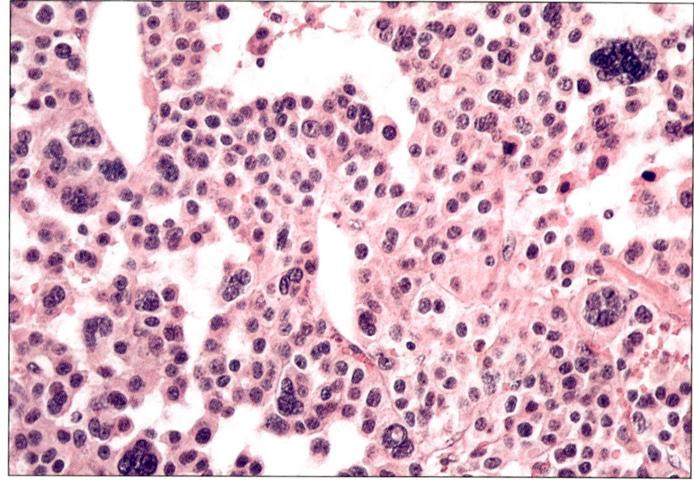

Figure 5.12 Leydig cell tumor. The nuclei are hyperchromatic and closely packed. Several giant, lobulated nuclei are present.

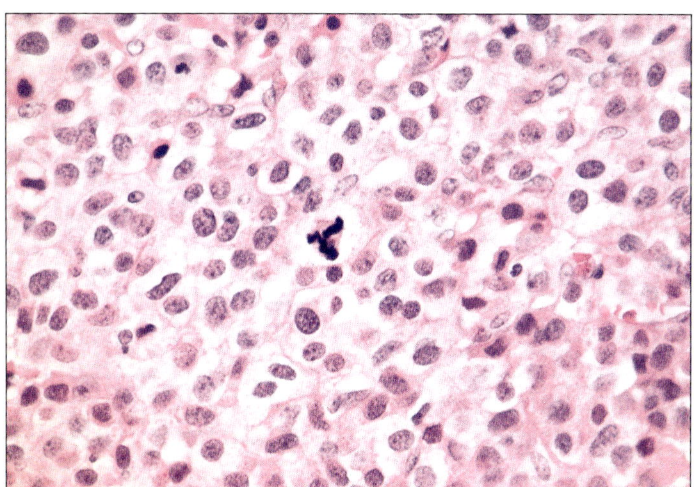

Figure 5.13 Leydig cell tumor. The nuclei are closely packed and moderately atypical. A tripolar mitotic figure is present.

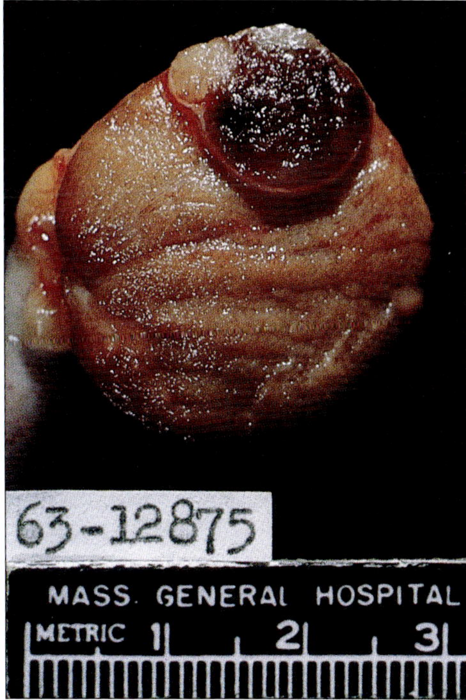

Figure 5.14 Sertoli cell tumor. The tumor is well circumscribed and exhibits extensive hemorrhage.

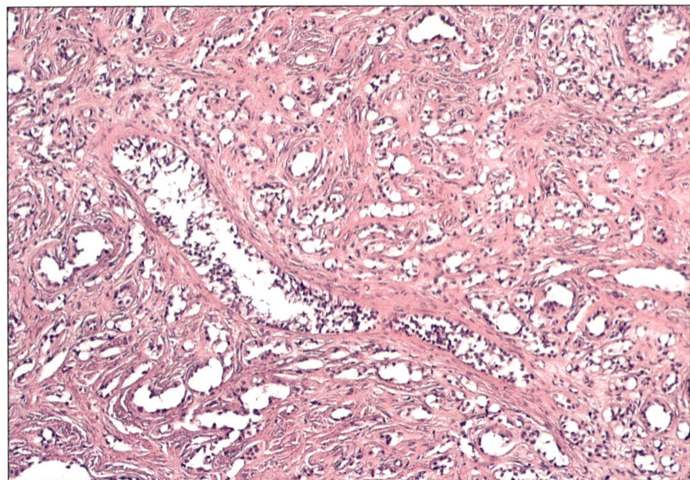

Figure 5.15 Sertoli cell tumor. The tumor is composed of tubules of varying sizes and shapes, which are mostly hollow, and smaller aggregates of neoplastic cells within a dense fibrous stroma.

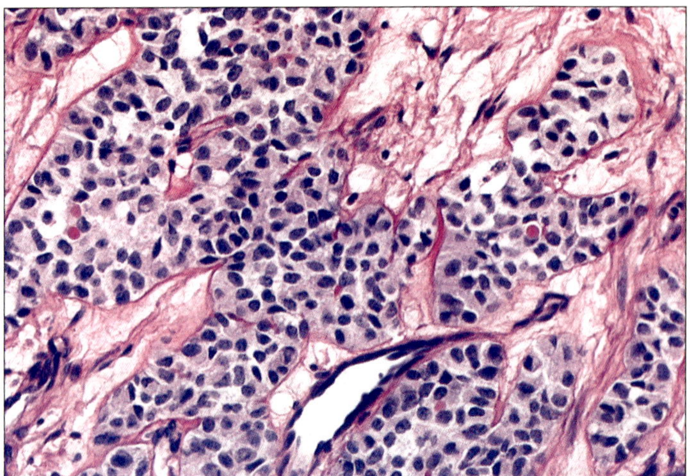

Figure 5.16 Sertoli cell tumor. The tumor cells are arranged in anastomosing, solid tubules and contain moderate amounts of cytoplasm and slightly atypical nuclei. Several intracellular hyaline bodies are present.

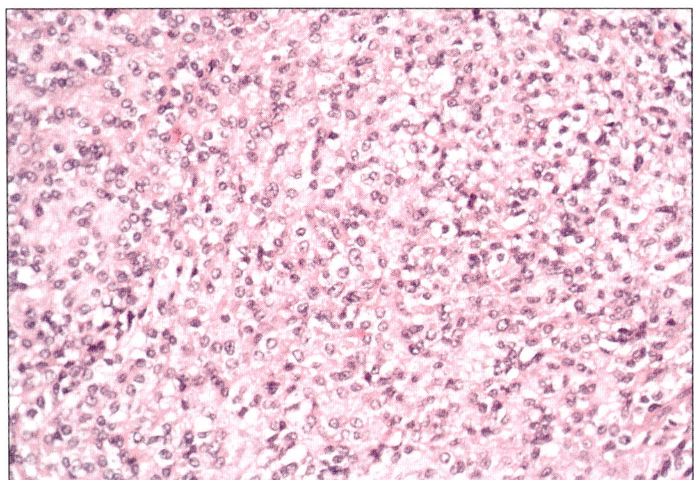

Figure 5.17 Sertoli cell tumor. The neoplastic cells are arranged diffusely and have cytoplasm that varies from eosinophilic to vacuolated and pale, and oval to round nuclei.

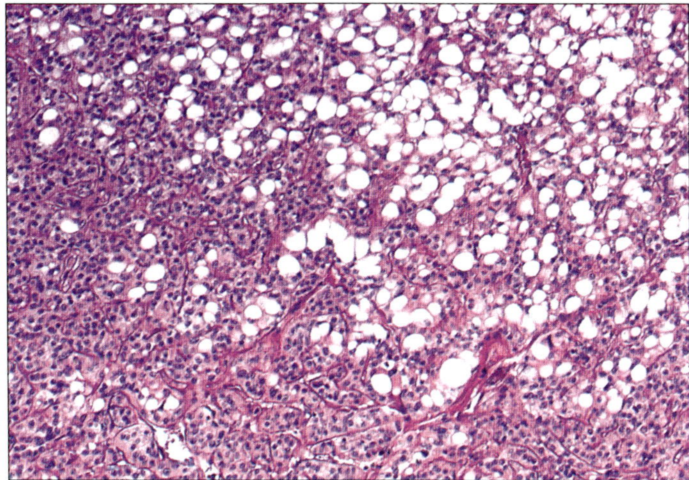

Figure 5.18 Sertoli cell tumor. The neoplastic cells are arranged in closely packed, small, solid tubules separated by delicate fibrovascular septa. Many of the cells contain large lipid vacuoles similar to those encountered in canine Sertoli cell tumors.

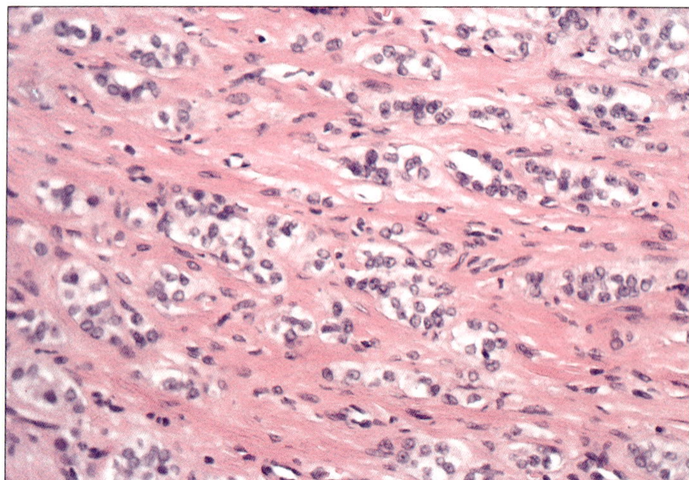

Figure 5.19 Sertoli cell tumor. The neoplastic cells are arranged in cords and small, solid, and hollow tubules separated by abundant hyalinized stroma.

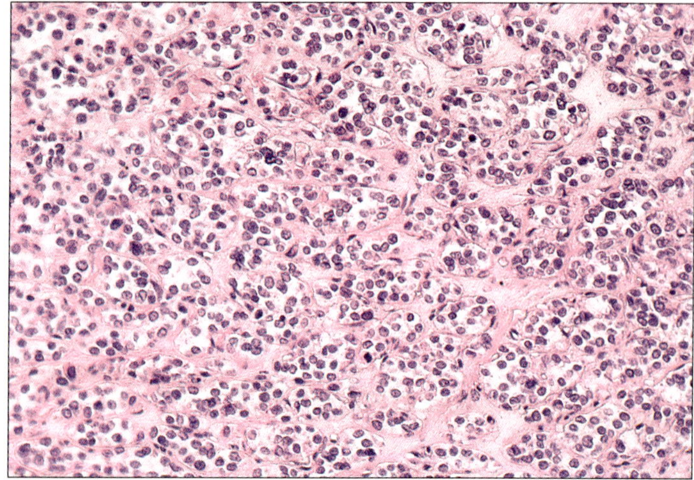

Figure 5.20 Sertoli cell tumor. This tumor, which metastasized, is composed of small, solid tubules separated by hypocellular connective tissue. The nuclei of the neoplastic cells are slightly atypical.

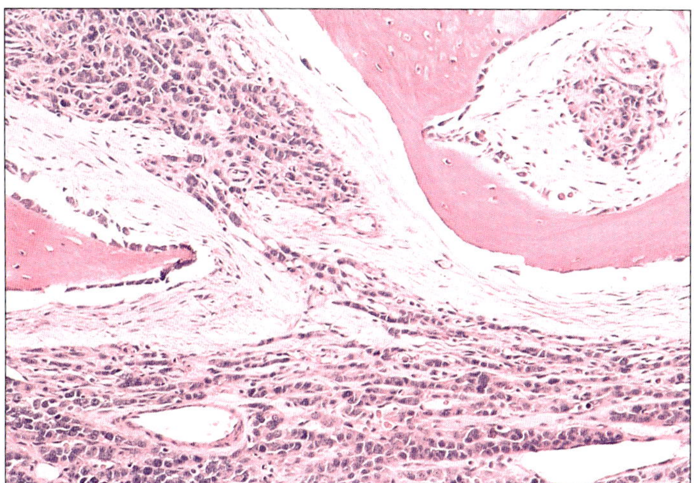

Figure 5.21 Sertoli cell tumor, metastatic to bone. This tumor, from the same patient whose primary tumor is illustrated in the preceding figure, is made up of closely packed cords of cells containing moderately atypical nuclei.

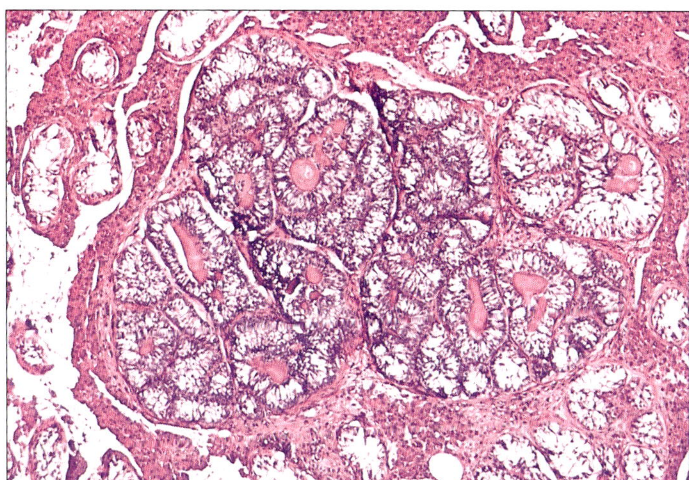

Figure 5.22 Sertoli cell nodule. This lobulated nodule, which was in a cryptorchid testis, is composed of small tubules filled with immature Sertoli cells. Some of the tubules are annular with central hyaline masses made up of basement membrane material.

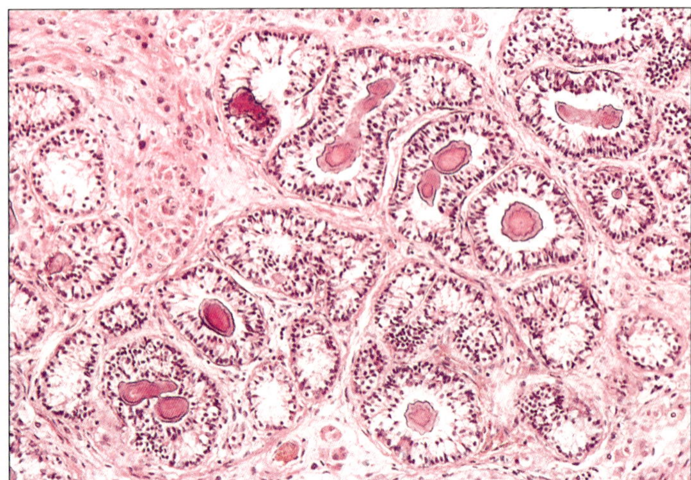

Figure 5.23 Sertoli cell nodule. This irregular nodule, which was in a cryptorchid testis, is made up of tubules containing immature Sertoli cells. Many of the tubules are annular and contain central laminated, calcific deposits.

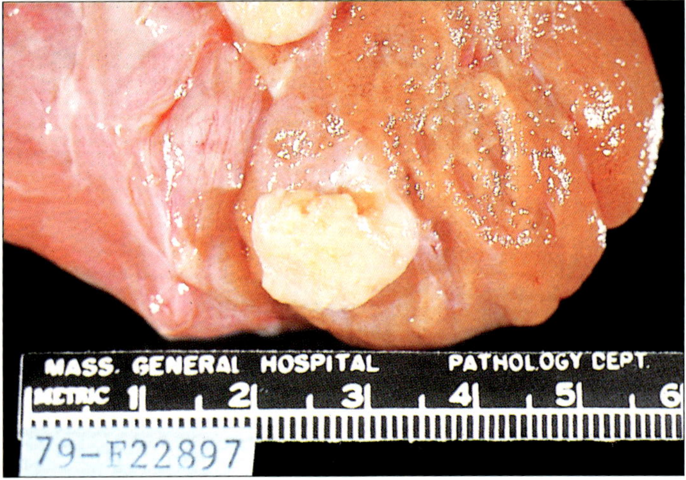

Figure 5.24 Large cell calcifying Sertoli cell tumor. The tumor is well demarcated and very pale yellow.

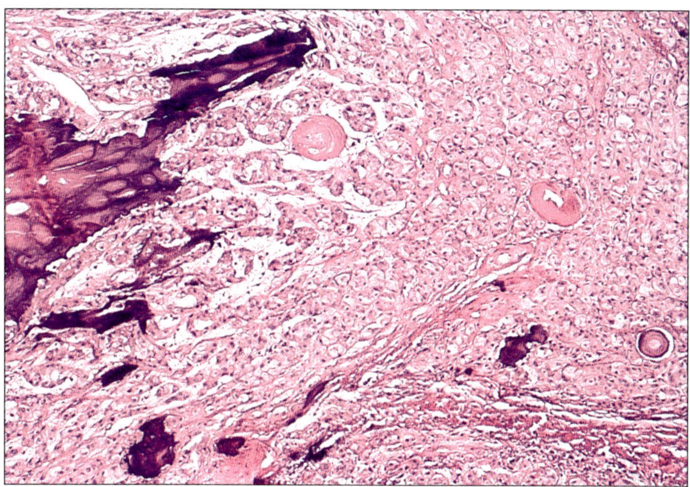

Figure 5.25 Large cell calcifying Sertoli cell tumor. The neoplastic cells are arranged diffusely and in small nests and trabeculae. There are numerous irregular aggregates of calcium as well as a small, round, laminated, calcified focus.

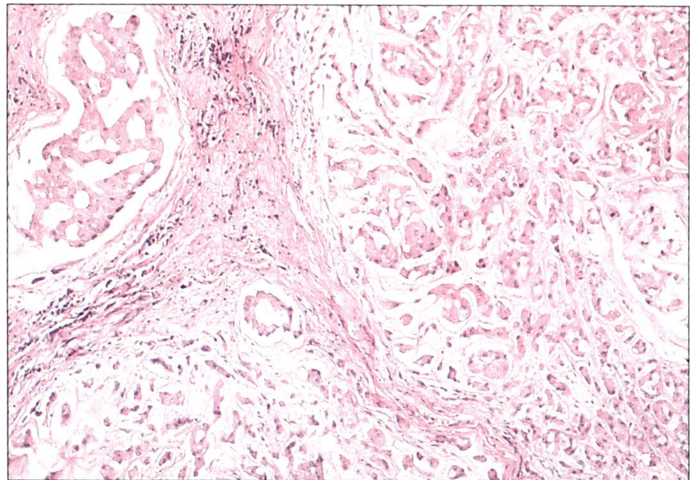

Figure 5.26 Large cell calcifying Sertoli cell tumor. The neoplastic cells are arranged in aggregates of varying sizes and shapes separated by myxoid stroma.

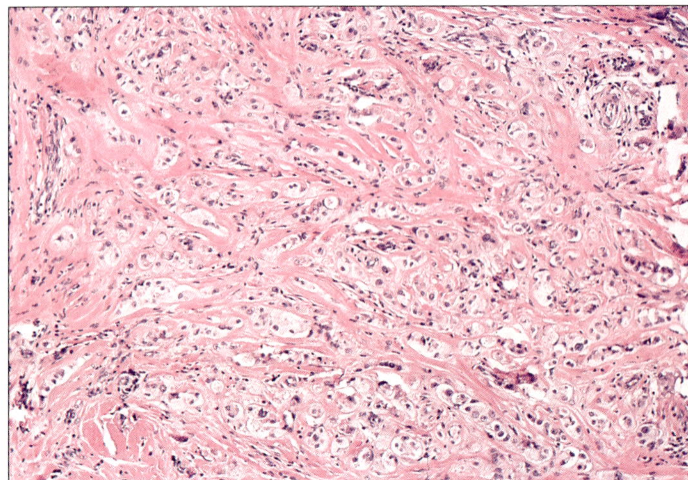

Figure 5.27 Large cell calcifying Sertoli cell tumor. Small clusters of neoplastic cells are separated by abundant fibrous stroma.

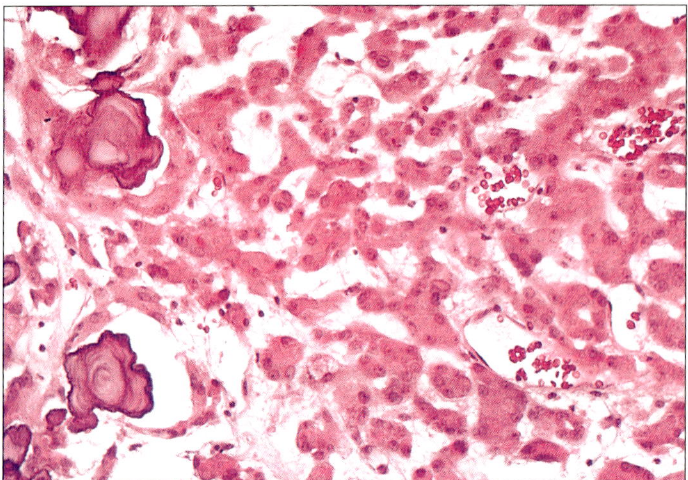

Figure 5.28 Large cell calcifying Sertoli cell tumor. The tumor cells contain abundant eosinophilic cytoplasm. Several laminated foci of calcification are present.

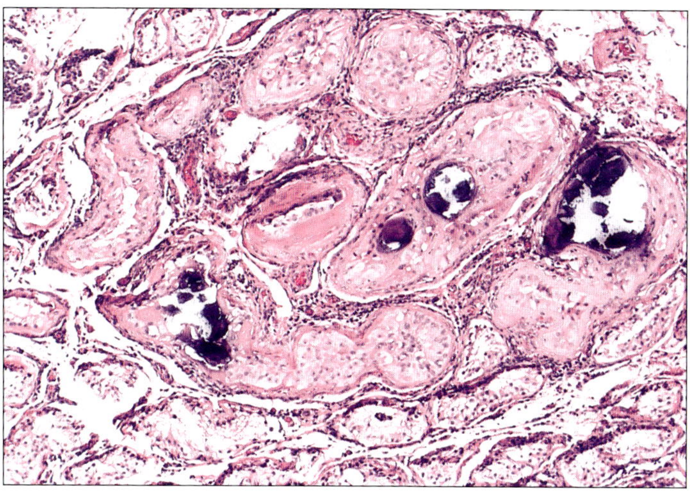

Figure 5.29 Large cell calcifying Sertoli cell tumor, intratubular. A cluster of tubules distended by focally calcified tumor is present.

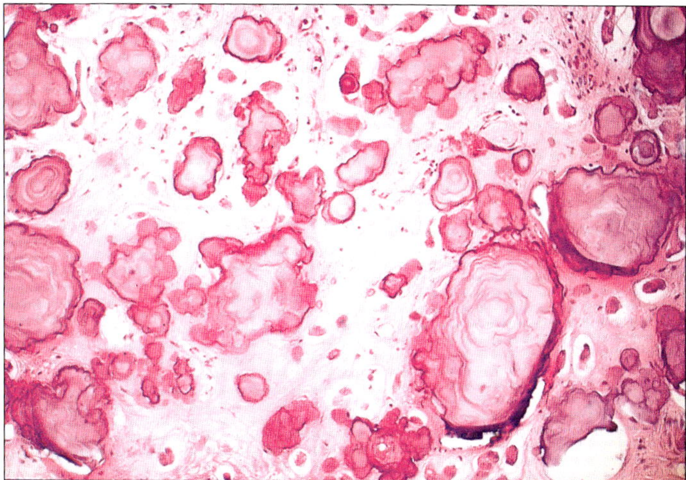

Figure 5.30 Large cell calcifying Sertoli cell tumor. This area of the tumor is almost entirely replaced by hyalinized connective tissue containing large numbers of wavy, laminated, calcific bodies of varying sizes and shapes.

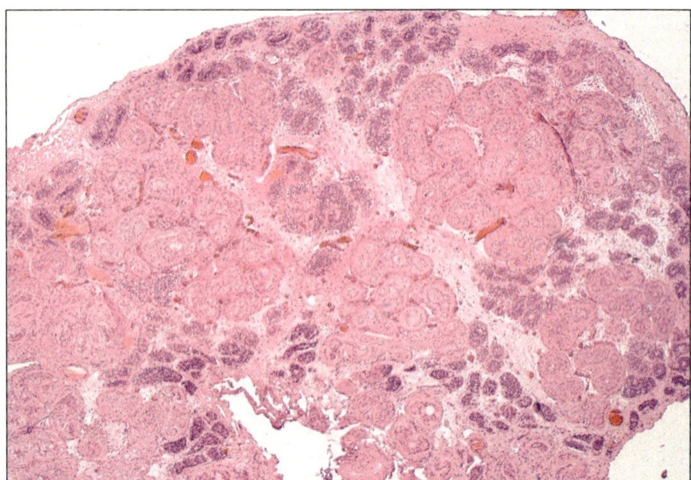

Figure 5.31 Large cell Sertoli cell tumor in Peutz-Jeghers syndrome. Most of the tubules are distended by neoplastic cells. No calcification was present in the tumor.

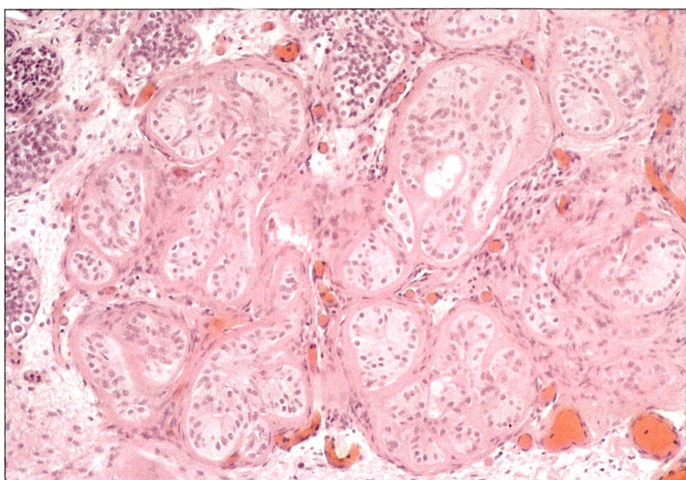

Figure 5.32 Large cell Sertoli cell tumor in Peutz-Jeghers syndrome. Most of the tubules are distended by neoplastic cells with abundant eosinophilic cytoplasm.

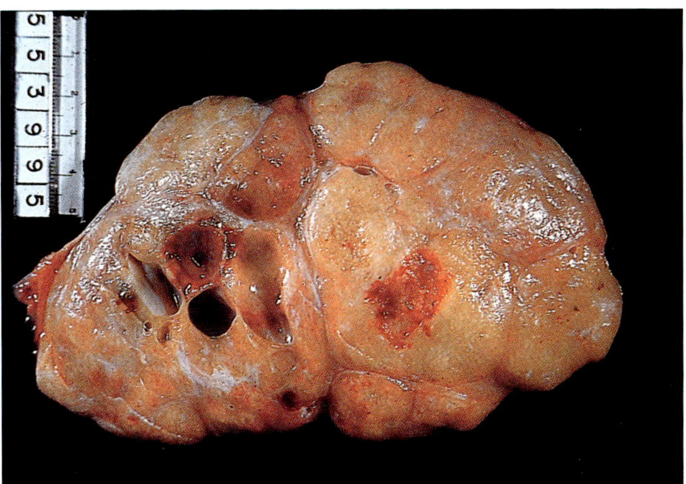

Figure 5.33 Granulosa cell tumor, adult type. The tumor is lobulated, brownish-yellow, and mostly solid, with focal hemorrhage.

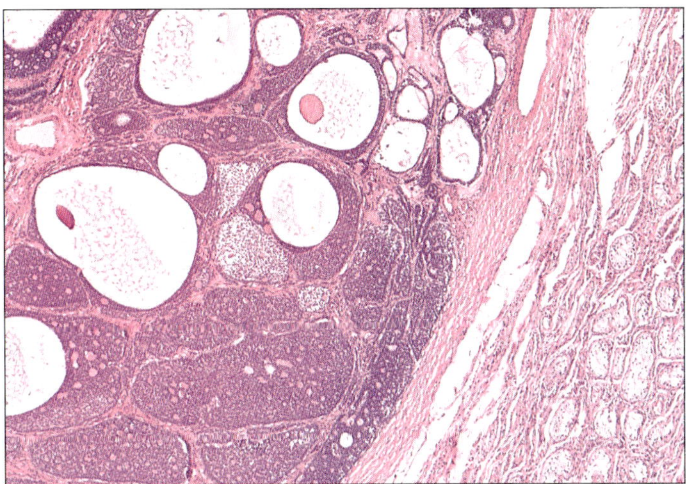

Figure 5.34 Granulosa cell tumor, adult type. The tumor contains Call-Exner bodies and larger follicles. (Courtesy of Dr Aleksander Talerman.)

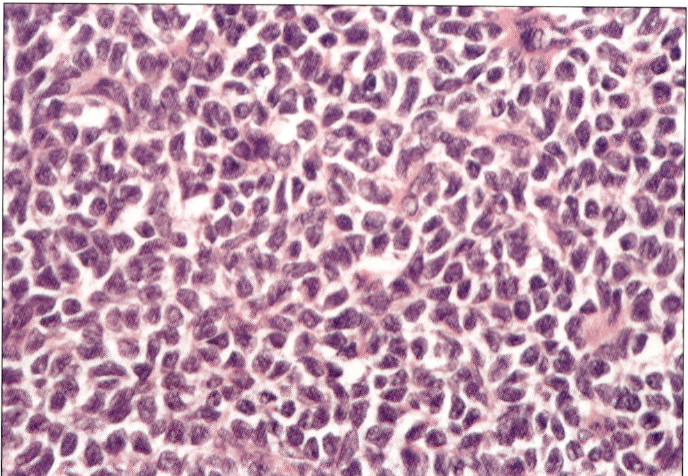

Figure 5.35 Granulosa cell tumor. The neoplastic cells have a diffuse pattern. They contain scanty cytoplasm and angular nuclei.

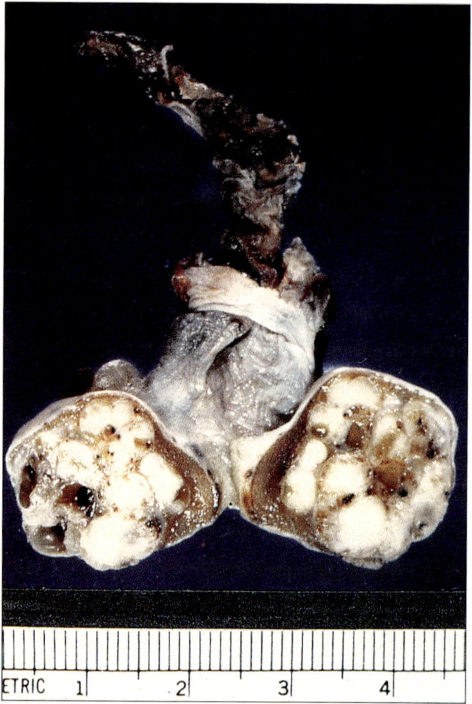

Figure 5.36 Juvenile granulosa cell tumor composed of multiple irregular, white nodules, and several cysts.

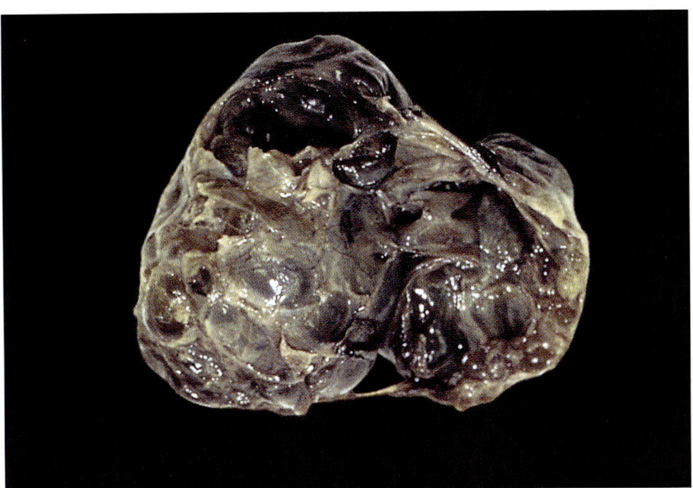

Figure 5.37 Juvenile granulosa cell tumor. The tumor is composed mainly of thin-walled cysts, some of which contain clotted blood.

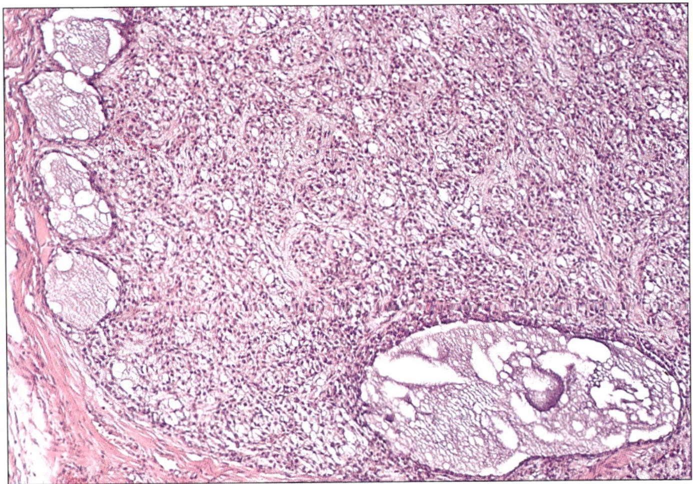

Figure 5.38 Juvenile granulosa cell tumor. The neoplastic cells are arranged diffusely and also form five follicles containing basophilic mucinous fluid.

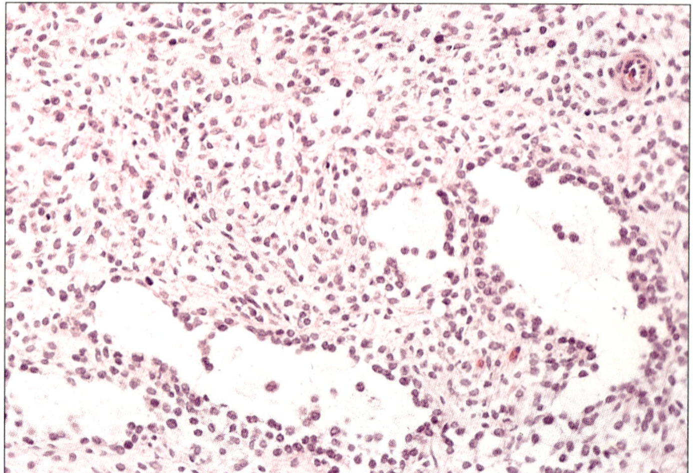

Figure 5.39 Juvenile granulosa cell tumor. Most of the neoplastic cells are arranged diffusely, but several follicles, varying in size and shape, contain pale basophilic fluid.

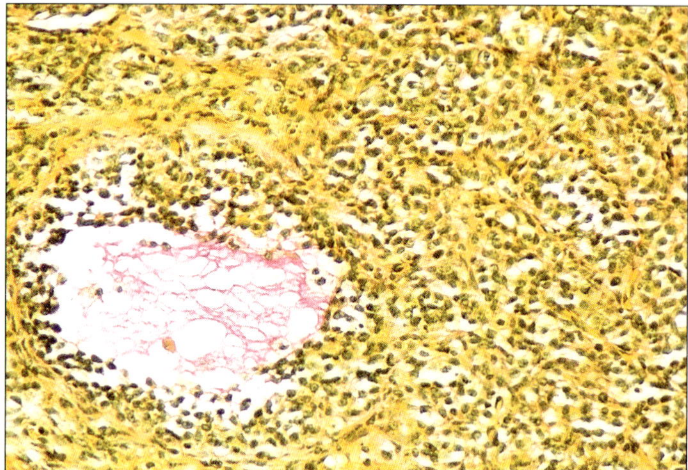

Figure 5.40 Juvenile granulosa cell tumor. The fluid in a follicle contains mucin stained by mucicarmine.

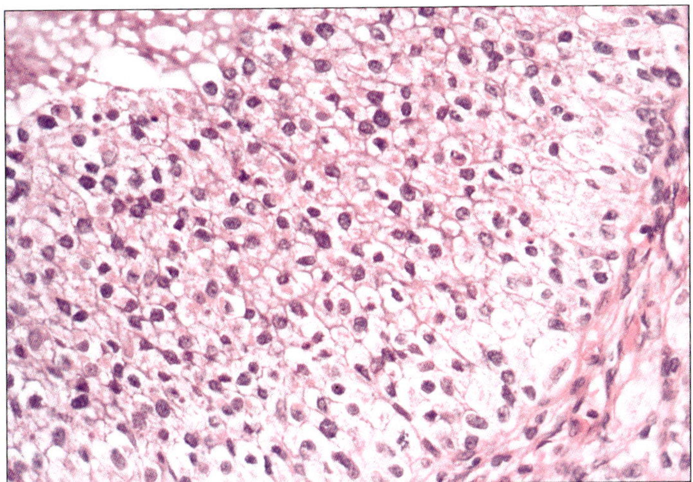

Figure 5.41 Juvenile granulosa cell tumor. The neoplastic cells are polyhedral to rounded and contain abundant cytoplasm and slightly atypical, rounded nuclei.

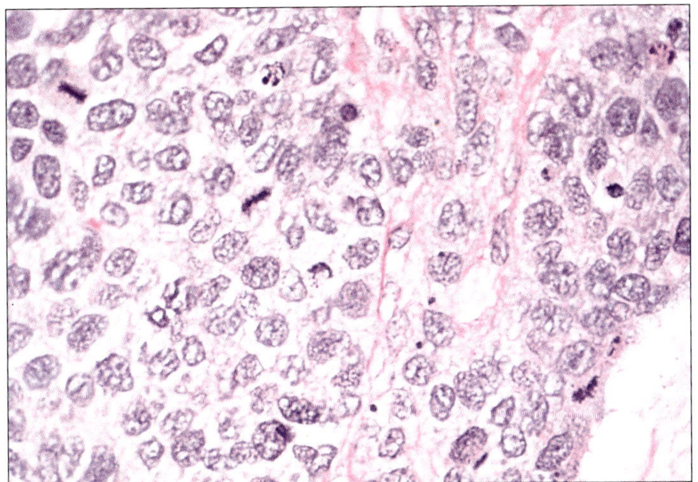

Figure 5.42 Juvenile granulosa cell tumor. The nuclei are atypical, and several mitotic figures are present.

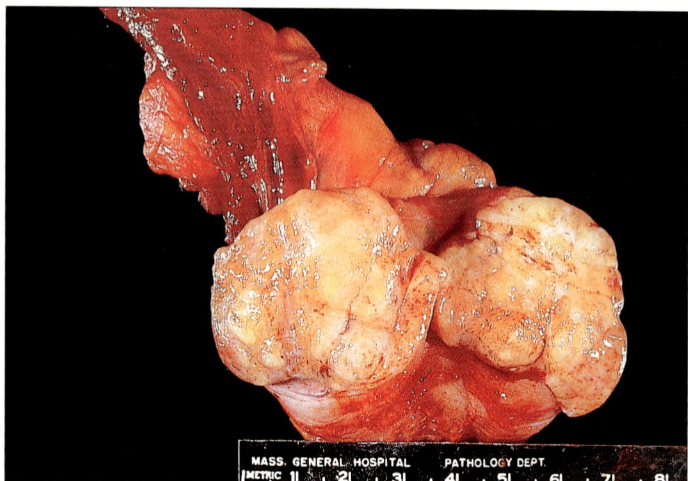

Figure 5.43 Sex cord–stromal tumor, unclassified. The tumor is pale yellow and lobulated.

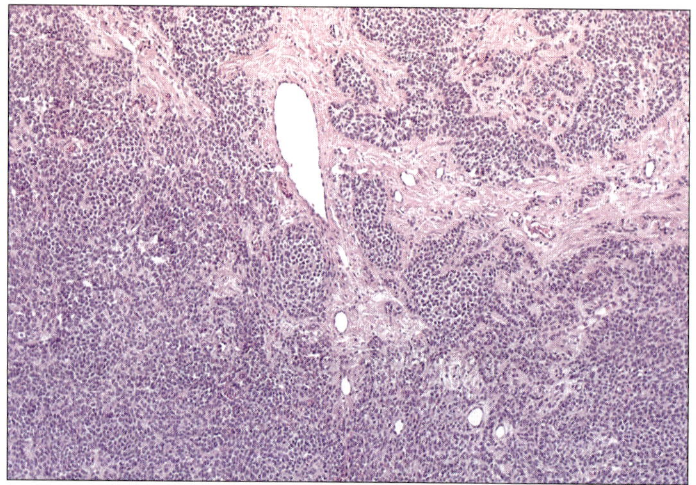

Figure 5.44 Sex cord–stromal tumor, unclassified. The tumor cells are arranged diffusely and in discrete aggregates.

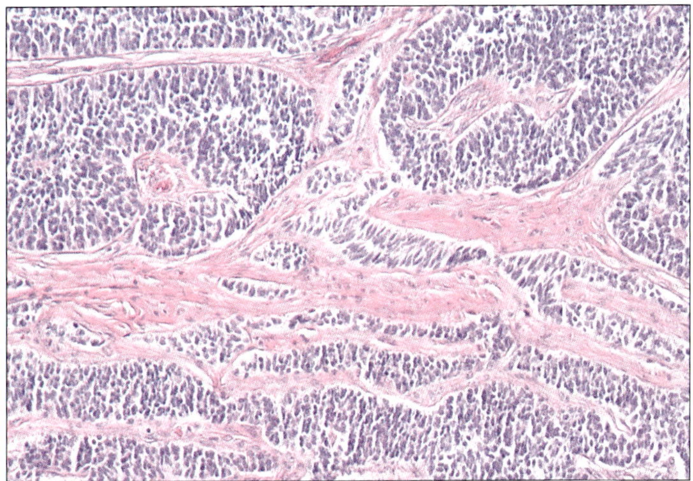

Figure 5.45 Sex cord-stromal tumor, unclassified. The tumor cells are arranged in anastomosing trabeculae and nests separated by abundant hypocellular fibrous stroma.

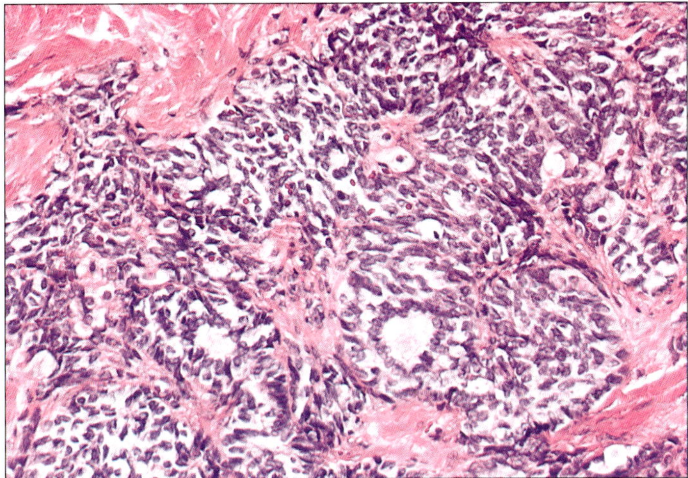

Figure 5.46 Sex cord–stromal tumor, unclassified. Anastomosing aggregates of tumor cells with spindle–shaped nuclei are arranged diffusely with a few structures resembling Call-Exner bodies, which contain pale eosinophilic fluid.

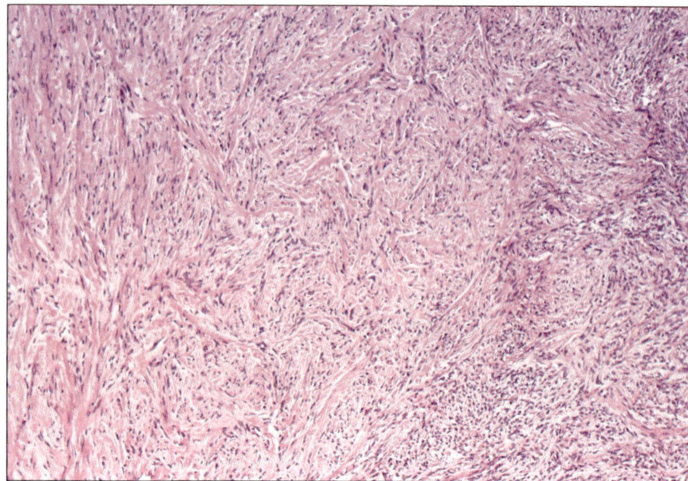

Figure 5.47 Sex cord–stromal tumor, unclassified. This portion of the tumor has an appearance resembling that of an ovarian fibroma.

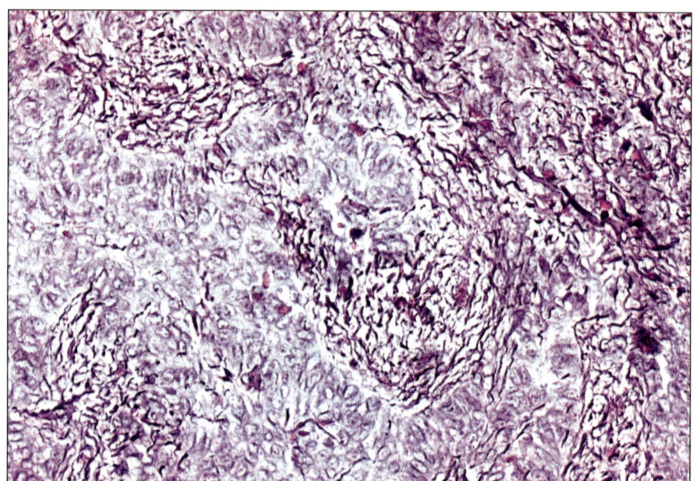

Figure 5.48 Sex cord–stromal tumor, unclassified. A reticulum stain demonstrates almost no fibrils within the sex cord component of the tumor and an abundant network in the stromal component.

References

1. Mostofi FK, Theiss EA, Ashley DJB. Tumors of specialized gonadal stroma in human male subjects. *Cancer* 12:944–957, 1959.
2. Lawrence WD, Young RH, Scully RE. Sex cord–stromal tumors. In: *Pathology of the Testis and its Adnexa*, Talerman A, Roth LM, eds. *Contemporary Issues in Surgical Pathology*, vol 7. New York, Churchill Livingstone, 1986, chap 4.
3. Kim I, Young RH, Scully RE. Leydig cell tumors of the testis: A clinicopathological analysis of 40 cases and review of the literature. *Am J Surg Pathol* 9:177–192, 1985.
4. Minokowitz S, Soloway H, Soscia J. Ossifying interstitial cell tumor of the testis. *J Urol* 94:592–595, 1965.
5. Scully RE, Coffin DL. Canine testicular tumors with special reference to their histogenesis, comparative morphology and endocrinology. *Cancer* 5:592–605, 1952.
6. Teilum G. Arrhenoblastoma-androblastoma; homologous ovarian and testicular tumors: II. Including so-called 'luteomas' and 'adrenal tumors' of ovary and interstitial cell tumors of testis. *Acta Pathol Microbiol Scand* 23:252–264, 1946.
7. Teilum G. Estrogen producing Sertoli-cell tumors (androblastoma tubulare lipoides of the human testis and ovary): Homologous ovarian and testicular tumors, III. *J Clin Endocrinol* 9:301–318, 1949.
8. Cantu JM, Rivera H, Ocampo-Campos R, et al. Peutz-Jeghers syndrome with feminizing Sertoli cell tumor. *Cancer* 46:223–228, 1980.
9. Dubois RS, Hoffman WH, Krishnan TH, et al. Feminizing sex cord tumor with annular tubules in a boy with Peutz-Jeghers syndrome. *J Pediatr* 101:568–571, 1982.
10. Ceccame AA, Cozzi F, Farragiana T, et al. Feminizing Sertoli cell tumor associated with Peutz-Jeghers syndrome. *Tumori* 71:379–385, 1985.
11. Wilson DM, Pitts WC, Hintz RL, Rosenfeld RG. Testicular tumors with Peutz-Jeghers syndrome. *Cancer* 57:2238–2240, 1986.
12. Young RH, Welch WR, Dickersin GR, Scully RE. Ovarian sex cord tumor with annular tubules: Review of 74 cases including 27 with Peutz-Jeghers syndrome and four with adenoma malignum of the cervix. *Cancer* 50:1384–1402, 1982.
13. Hedinger CE, Huber R, Weber E. Frequency of so-called hypoplastic or dysgenetic zones in scrotal and otherwise normal human testes. *Virchows Arch A* 342:165–168, 1967.
14. Proppe KH, Scully RE: Large-cell calcifying Sertoli cell tumor of the testis. *Am J Clin Pathol* 74:607–619, 1980.
15. Carney JA, Gordon H, Carpenter PC, et al. The complex of myxomas, spotty pigmentation, and endocrine overactivity. *Medicine* 64:270–283, 1985.
16. Waxman M, Damjanov I, Khapra A, Landal SJ: Large cell calcifying Sertoli tumor of testis: Light microscopic and ultrastructural study. *Cancer* 54:1574–1581, 1984.

17. Horn T, Jao W, Keh PC. Large-cell calcifying Sertoli cell tumor of the testis: A case report with ultrastructural study. *Ultrastruct Pathol* 4:359–364, 1983.
18. Talerman A. Pure granulosa cell tumor of the testis: Report of a case and review of the literature. *Appl Pathol* 3:117–122, 1985.
19. Gaylis FD, August C, Yeldandi A, et al. Granulosa cell tumor of the adult testis: Ultrastructural and ultrasonographic characteristics. *J Urol* 141:126–127, 1989.
20. Crump WD. Juvenile granulosa cell (sex cord–stromal) tumor of fetal testis. *J Urol* 129:1057–1058, 1983.
21. Lawrence WD, Young RH, Scully RE. Juvenile granulosa cell tumor of the infantile testis: A report of fourteen cases. *Am J Surg Pathol* 9:87–94, 1985.
22. Young RH, Lawrence WD, Scully RE. Juvenile granulosa cell tumor: Another neoplasm associated with abnormal chromosomes and ambiguous genitalia: A report of three cases. *Am J Surg Pathol* 9:737–743, 1985.
23. Raju U, Fine G, Warrier R, et al. Congenital testicular juvenile granulosa cell tumor in a patient with x/xy mosaicism. *Am J Surg Pathol* 10:577–583, 1986.
24. Rosvoll RV, Woodard JR. Malignant Sertoli cell tumor of the testis. *Cancer* 22:8–13, 1968.
25. Kaplan GW, Cromie WJ, Kelalis PP, et al. Gonadal stromal tumors: A report of the prepubertal testicular tumor registry. *J Urol* 136:300–302, 1986.
26. Herrera LO, Wilk H, Wills JS, Lopez GE. Malignant (androblastoma) Sertoli cell tumor of testis. *Urology* 18:287–290, 1981.
27. Dauplat J, Dionet C, Ferriere JP, et al. Tumeur maligne du stroma gonadique testiculaire: Traitement par une association chimiothérapie-radiothérapie. *J Urol* 91:53–57, 1985.
28. Godec CJ. Malignant Sertoli cell tumor of testicle. *Urology* 26:185–188, 1985.
29. Gabrilove JL, Freiberg, EK, Leiter E, Nicolis GL. Feminizing and nonfeminizing Sertoli cell tumors. *J Urol* 124:757–767, 1980.

6 Tumors and Tumorlike Lesions in Intersexual Disorders

Although most patients with intersexual disorders are raised as females, some of them are phenotypically male. In either case, if their gonads contain testicular tissue, it is unusually susceptible to neoplasia as well as the development of tumorlike lesions.[1,2] The three most common disorders of sexual development that merit consideration in this regard are mixed gonadal dysgenesis, true hermaphroditism, and the androgen insensitivity syndrome.

Mixed Gonadal Dysgenesis

In this disorder, there may be a streak composed of ovarian-type stroma on one side and a testis on the other side or unilateral or bilateral streak testes.[3] The phenotype is usually female, with varying degrees of masculinization of the secondary sex organs in most of the cases; in other subjects the phenotype is male, but the external genitalia are incompletely masculinized in the majority of these cases. In some patients, the virilization of the external genitalia is asymmetric. A rare disorder closely related to mixed gonadal dysgensis is dysgenetic male pseudohermaphroditism, in which bilateral poorly developed testes are present; its clinical and pathological features merge almost imperceptibly with those of mixed gonadal dysgenesis. Patients with mixed gonadal dysgenesis most commonly have a 45X, 46XY karyotype.

The testis in mixed gonadal dysgenesis ranges from a well-developed to an immature testis that may contain misshapen, branching tubules and ovarian-type stroma. In a streak testis, the streak tissue is typically peripheral to the testicular tissue.

Two lesions exist in the testes and streak testes of patients with mixed gonadal dysgenesis that may be precursors of invasive germ cell tumors: intratubular germ cell neoplasia, unclassified (IGCNU)[4] (see Chapter 4) and gonadoblastoma.[5] In one investigation of testicular changes in four children with mixed gonadal dysgenesis, 1 month to 17 years of age, IGCNU was found in all cases.[4]

The gonadoblastoma (Figures 6.1 to 6.4), which occurs mainly in patients with mixed gonadal dysgenesis, 46XY pure gonadal dysgenesis (bilateral streak gonads with failure of development of secondary sex organs and characteristics), and dysgenetic male pseudohermaphroditism, is a mixed tumor composed of germ cells resembling seminoma cells, small round to rod-shaped cells, which are immature Sertoli cells and may contain Charcot-Böttcher filament bundles,[6] and, in two thirds of the cases, steroid-type cells, which are probably Leydig cells. The germ cells and sex cord elements are typically present in rounded to irregular discrete nests in one or more of three patterns. Most characteristically the sex cord cells surround rounded hyaline nodules of basement membrane material (Figures 6.2, 6.4) and often merge with the basement membrane surrounding the nest. Second, the sex cord cells may have a coronal relation to the germ cells (Figures 6.2, 6.3), resembling follicular epithelium surrounding an ovum, and third, the sex cord cells may form a ring of single cells at the periphery of the nest with a germ cell population at the center. In occasional cases, both germ cells and sex cord cells grow diffusely. Most gonadoblastomas exhibit focal to extensive calcification (Figure 6.2), which typically begins in the hyaline bodies and may in some cases form large, wavy, laminated masses separated by dense fibrous tissue. The Leydig-like cells, which are seen more commonly after the onset of puberty, appear as aggregates of large polyhedral cells lacking crystals of Reinke (Figure 6.4).

Gonadoblastomas have ranged in diameter from microscopic to 8 cm. When grossly detectable, they are composed of pale yellow to cream-colored tissue, which may be flecked with calcific deposits or be massively calcified. The gonadoblastoma itself can be viewed as an in situ germ cell tumor lacking a capacity to spread beyond the gonad. It is impossible to state accurately how often a testicular gonadoblastoma is the source of an invasive germ cell tumor because the latter may obliterate evidence of the former and most gonadoblastomas have already replaced the gonads in which they arose, making identification of the nature of the gonad impossible. If, however, one considers gonadoblastomas of testicular, streak, and unknown gonadal origins collectively, approximately one half of those that remain detectable are associated with invasive germinoma (seminoma or dysgerminoma) and 8% are associated with a germ cell tumor of another type such as embryonal carcinoma, yolk sac tumor, or teratoma. Gonadoblastomas and pure germ cell tumors are said to develop in 25% of patients with mixed gonadal dysgenesis by the age of 40 years.[7]

Lesions that must be distinguished from gonadoblastomas include the small, nonneoplastic nodules composed of immature Sertoli cells that occur primarily in cryptorchid testes when such nodules contain germ cells, and the very rare germ cell–sex cord–stromal tumors, unclassified. The former lesions, which are encountered almost exclusively in patients with normal sexual development, do not exhibit the variety of patterns characteristic of gonadoblastomas. Germ cell–sex cord–stromal tumors, unclassified also occur very rarely in the testes of otherwise normal males.[8,9] They may be intratubular or form invasive masses (Figure 6.5). The sex cord elements vary in their degree of maturity and the germ cells may have the appearance of seminoma cells or more mature germ cells. The tumor cells grow in tubular, trabecular, and diffuse patterns, but focally may exhibit patterns resembling those of gonadoblastoma. The stromal component, when present, is composed of cells resembling Leydig cells. A malignant germ cell neoplasm has not been reported to arise from a testicular tumor of this type, in contrast to the occurrence of germinomas and other germ cell tumors in cases of gonadoblastoma.

In addition to gonadoblastomas and germ cell tumors, juvenile granulosa cell tumors appear to occur more frequently in the testes of patients with mixed gonadal dysgenesis.[10]

True Hermaphroditism

In true hermaphroditism, there may be a testis on one side and an ovary on the other side, or unilateral or bilateral ovotestes.[11] The patients' phenotypes range from nomal female to normal male, but the majority of them are females with varying degrees of virilization. The most common karyotype is 46XX. Unlike mixed gonadal dysgenesis, true hermaphroditism is typically characterized by the presence of initially normal-appearing ovarian and testicular tissue. The ovary is physiologically dominant, ovulation and rarely pregnancy may occur, and the testis typically undergoes atrophy with tubular sclerosis. There appears to be an increased incidence of germ cell neoplasia of various types in true hermaphrodites. It is usually difficult to determine whether a large tumor has arisen in the ovarian or testicular tissue in these patients, but in view of the variety of gonadal tumors that have been reported in them, it is probable that any type of testicular or ovarian tumor may be encountered. Gonadoblastomas have also been described in true hermaphrodites, but the frequency of gonadoblastomas and pure germ cell tumors in such patients is under 3%.[11]

Androgen Insensitivity Syndrome

This syndrome, also designated testicular feminization, occurs in 46XY-phenotypic females with testes.[2] The testes, which are almost always abdominal, inguinal, or labial, secrete initially normal amounts of androgens, but the end-organs have defects in their receptor mechanism, resulting in an incomplete to complete lack of response to androgenic stimulation. The patients generally lack müllerian duct derivatives because testicular secretion of müllerian inhibiting substance results in complete or almost complete inhibition of müllerian duct development; fallopian tubes, however, are occasionally present. The disease may be familial, with varying numbers of sisters and maternal aunts affected. The patient with the complete form of the syndrome may come to the attention of the physician because of a family history of the disorder, a femoral hernia during childhood, primary amenorrhea because of absence of a uterus, or the development of a gonadal tumor or tumorlike lesion, usually after the age of puberty.

The testes in the complete androgen insensitivity syndrome are of almost normal size and are attached medially to muscular cords, which may be hypertrophied gubernacula, and laterally to adnexal structures, which are often cystic. The testicular parenchyma is dark brown and may be flecked with small yellow foci. Microscopic examination reveals three components, which vary in prominence and may undergo changes with increasing age: tubules, Leydig cells, and stroma resembling ovarian stroma (Figures 6.6 to 6.10). The tubules are smaller than normal and are composed predominantly of immature Sertoli cells (Figure 6.6); rare to occasional spermatogonia may be scattered along their basement membranes (Figure 6.8). After puberty, some of the tubules may enlarge, with some degree of maturation of the Sertoli cells. With increasing age, the tubules may undergo atrophy with sclerosis, which may be extensive and obscure the nature of the gonad. The Leydig cells are generally robust after the age of puberty and are usually diffusely or focally hyperplastic (Figures 6.6, 6.7). They may be few and scattered in old patients; crystals of Reinke are rarely present. Stroma resembling ovarian stroma may be absent or may be the predominant stromal component (Figure 6.9); it may contain individual steroid-type cells or small nests of them (Figure 6.10). When the stromal component predominates and few tubules are present, the gonad may be mistaken for an ovary.

Beginning in the teenage years, hamartomatous nodules, which are composed of the various cellular constituents of the gonad, appear in the testes of as many as one fourth of patients with the complete androgen insensitivity syndrome. These lesions are usually multiple and typically are up to 5 cm in diameter; depending on their predominant cellular constituents, their sectioned surfaces range from white to yellow-brown (Figures 6.11, 6.12). These hamartomas are usually made up predominantly of solid tubules lined by immature Sertoli cells and separated by Leydig cells in varying amounts (Figure 6.13); scattered spermatogonia may be present within the tubules. A rare hamartoma is composed predominantly of stroma resembling ovarian stroma and has the microscopic features of an ovarian fibroma.

Several types of tumor in the sex cord–stromal category occur in the testes of patients with the complete androgen insensitivity syndrome. The most common is a pure Sertoli cell tumor (Figure 6.14) made up of closely packed, strikingly uniform, solid tubules containing immature Sertoli cells (Figure 6.15). These tumors may attain diameters of 25 cm and typically are composed of firm white tissue. Much less common is a Leydig cell tumor. A few examples of malignant sex cord tumors have also been encountered.[12]

The most common serious neoplastic complication of the androgen insensitivity syndrome is the development of a malignant germ cell tumor, most commonly a seminoma (Figures 6.12, 6.16), but in occasional cases some other type of germ cell tumor. The precancerous lesion IGCNU has also been observed both before and after the age of puberty in three of 12 young patients with incomplete forms of the syndrome,[13] but gonadoblastomas have not been reported. A malignant germ cell tumor is said to develop in over 30% of patients with the complete form of the androgen insensitivity syndrome by the age of 50 years; such a tumor is extremely rare before the age of puberty.[7] It is unclear how much the increased frequency of germ cell neoplasia is related to cryptorchidism and how much is related to the abnormal sexual differentiation per se. Except for the above-mentioned cases of IGCNU and a single case of an invasive germ cell tumor,[14] there is no published evidence of an increased frequency of neoplasia in association with incomplete forms of androgen insensitivity syndrome, of which many fewer cases have been reported.

Finally, adnexal cysts of wolffian or müllerian origin may on occasion be large enough to result in palpable tumorlike masses. These cysts are typically multilocular and filled with clear fluid.

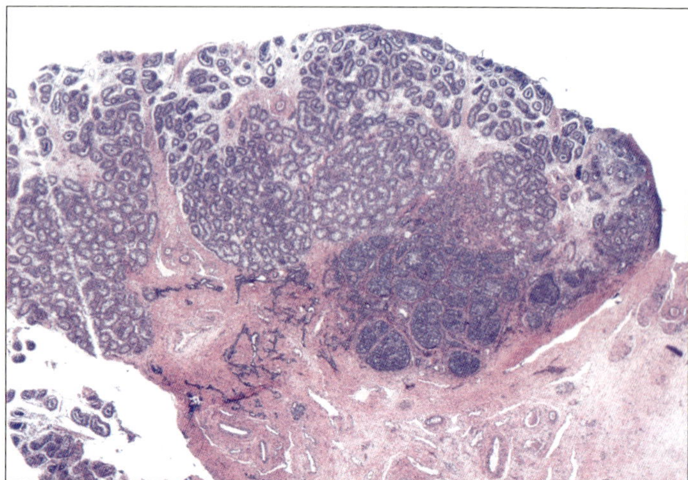

Figure 6.1 Gonadoblastoma. A small, rounded nodule made up of closely packed nests of gonadoblastoma is present to the right of the rete testis.

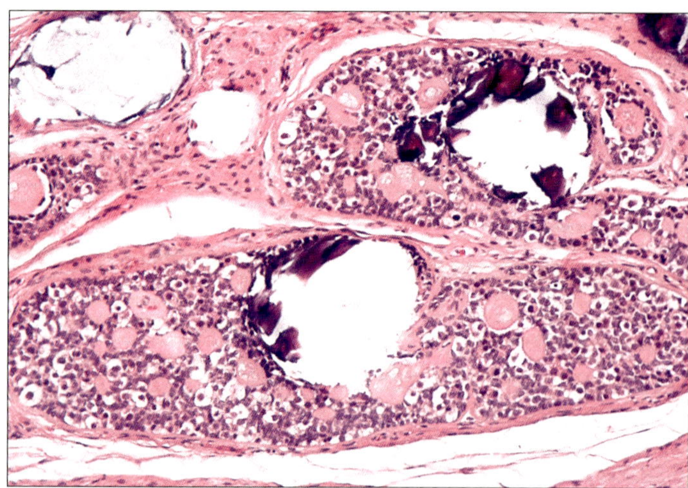

Figure 6.2 Gonadoblastoma. Several large nests are composed of large germ cells surrounded by numerous smaller cells of sex cord type. Numerous rounded nodules made up of basement membrane material and several calcified foci are present.

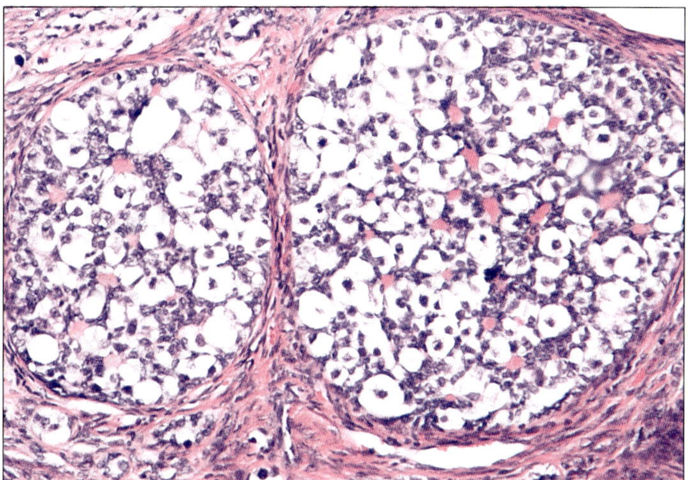

Figure 6.3 Gonadoblastoma. Two rounded nests are composed of large germinoma cells with abundant clear cytoplasm separated by smaller cells of sex cord type. Scattered small hyaline nodules made up of basement membrane material are also visible.

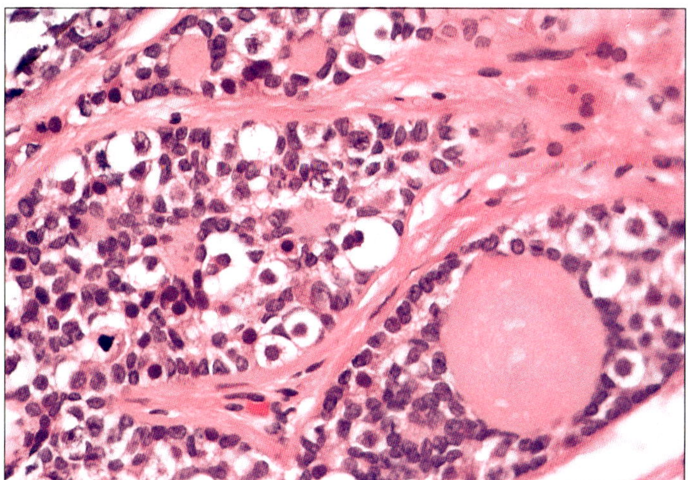

Figure 6.4 Gonadoblastoma. Several nodules of neoplastic cells are separated by dense fibrous tissue. A few cells containing abundant eosinophilic cytoplasm and resembling Leydig cells are present in the right upper corner of the photomicrograph. The germ cells resemble those of the seminoma and the smaller cells of sex cord type resemble immature Sertoli cells. Several hyalinized nodules made up of basement membrane material are also visible.

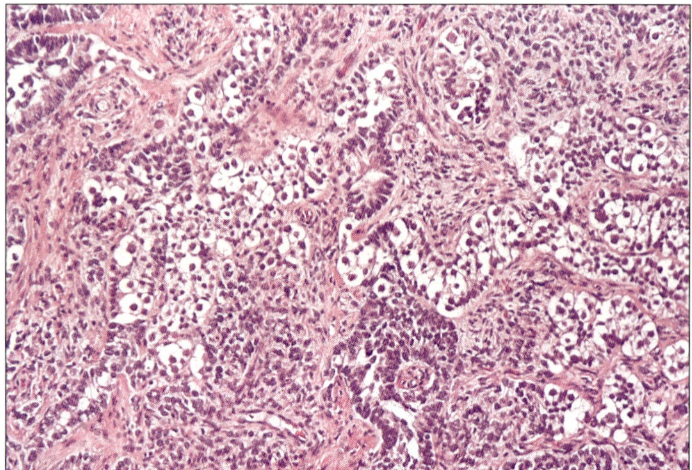

Figure 6.5 Germ cell–sex cord–stromal tumor, unclassified. Irregular nests and solid tubules made up of germ cells and sex cord–type cells are separated by cellular stroma. The germ cells contain abundant clear cytoplasm and central nuclei.

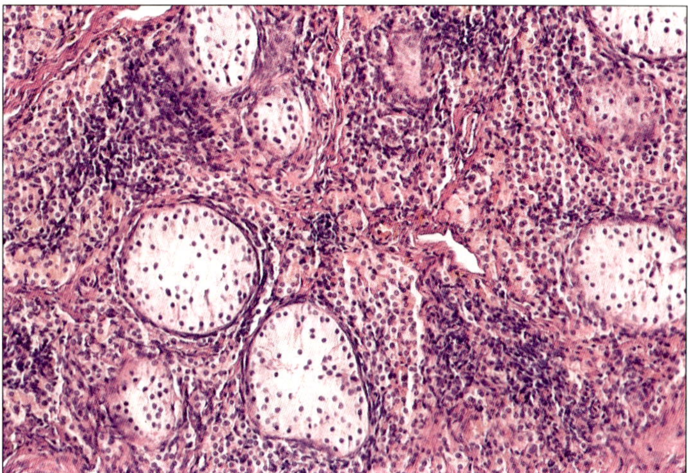

Figure 6.6 Testis in androgen insensitivity syndrome. Tubules containing Sertoli cells are widely separated by cellular stroma resembling ovarian stroma and large numbers of Leydig cells.

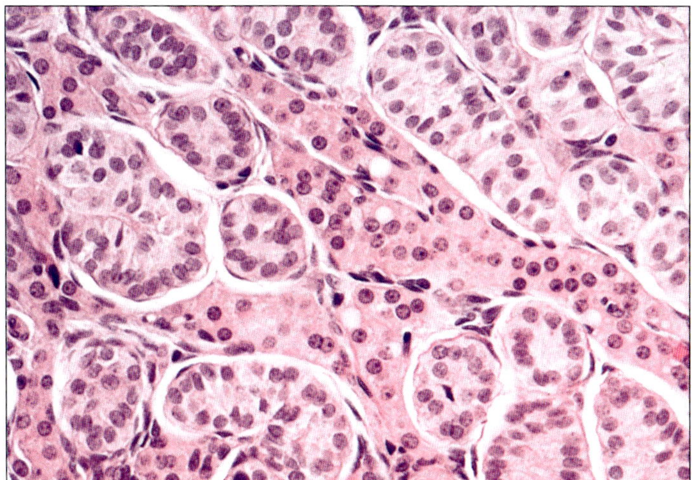

Figure 6.7 Testis in androgen insensitivity syndrome. Solid tubules containing Sertoli cells are separated by Leydig cells.

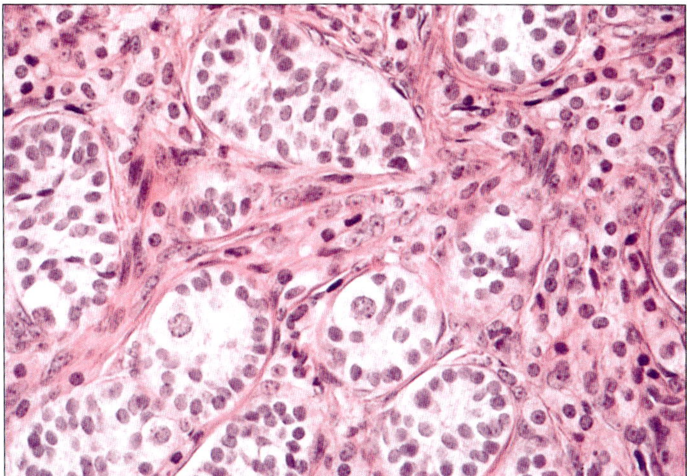

Figure 6.8 Testis in androgen insensitivity syndrome. Occasional large germ cells with prominent round nuclei are present within several of the tubules.

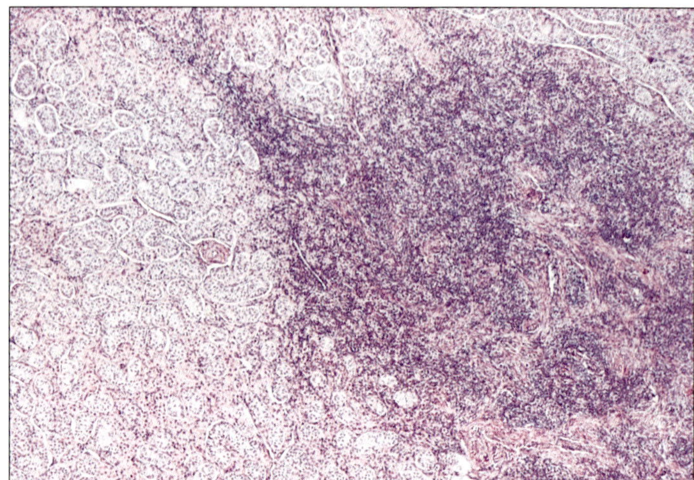

Figure 6.9 Testis in androgen insensitivity syndrome. The right portion of the photomicrograph is occupied by densely cellular stroma resembling ovarian stroma.

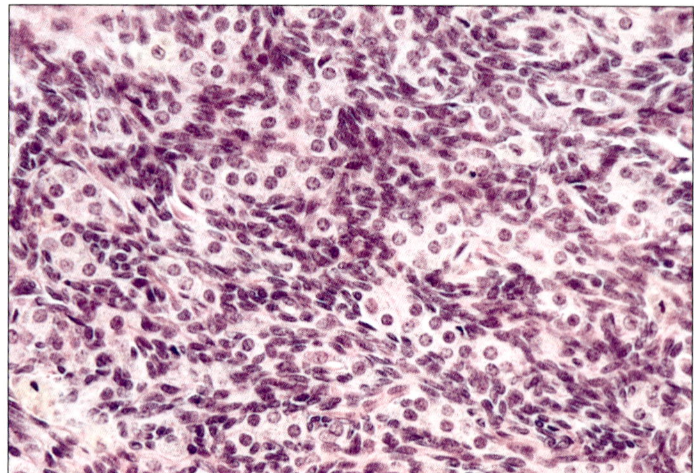

Figure 6.10 Testis in androgen insensitivity syndrome. Numerous Leydig cells are present in a background of stroma resembling ovarian stroma.

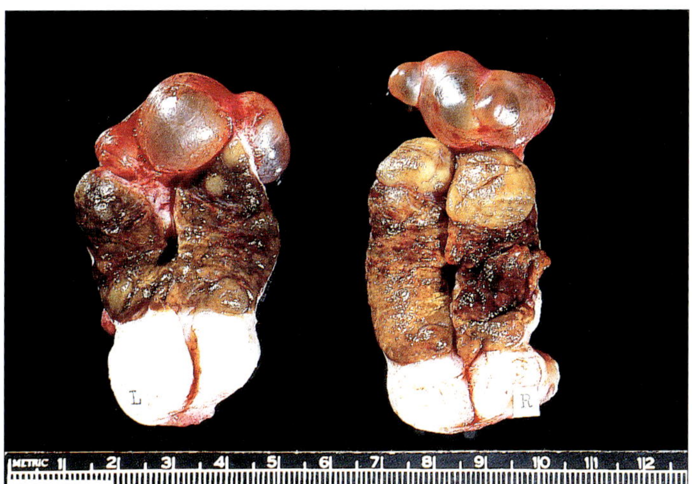

Figure 6.11 Hamartomas in testis of androgen insensitivity syndrome. The testes contain multiple bulging nodules ranging in color from pale yellow to light brown. Multilocular adnexal cysts are present at the upper (lateral) poles of the testes. White, rounded, smooth muscle bodies are present at the lower (medial) poles.

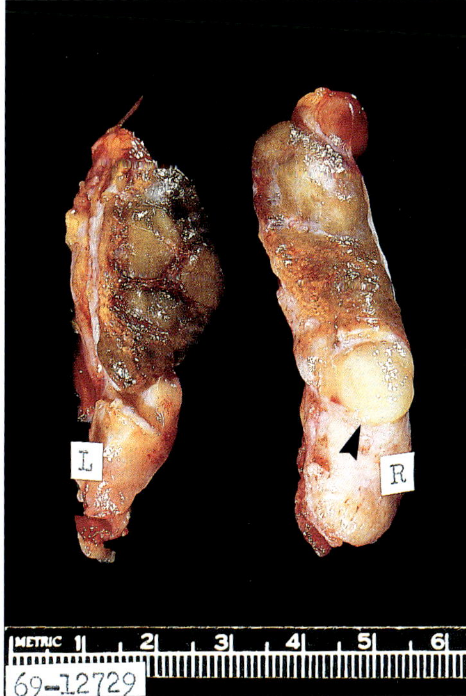

Figure 6.12 Seminoma (arrow) and hamartomas in testes of androgen insensitivity syndrome.

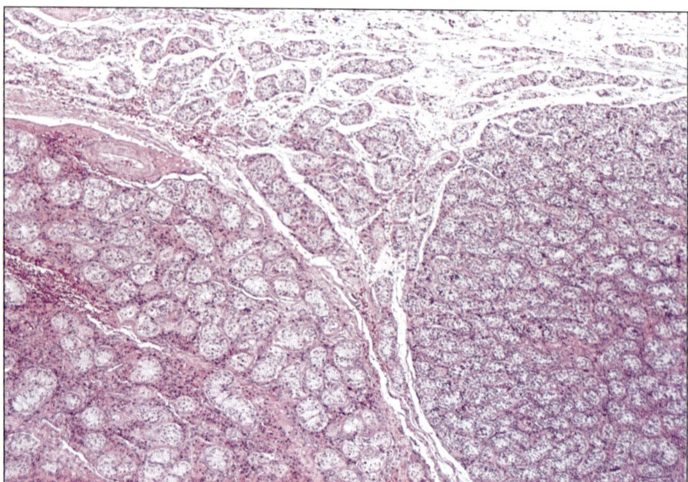

Figure 6.13 Hamartomas in testis of androgen insensitivity syndrome. Two rounded nodules are made up predominantly of closely packed tubules. The nodule on the left side also contains numerous Leydig cells.

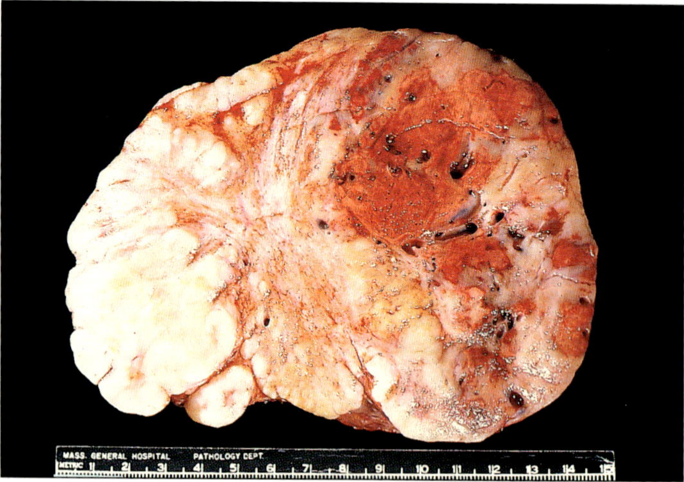

Figure 6.14 Sertoli cell adenoma in testis of androgen insensitivity syndrome. The neoplastic tissue is cream-colored and contains numerous foci of hemorrhage and necrosis.

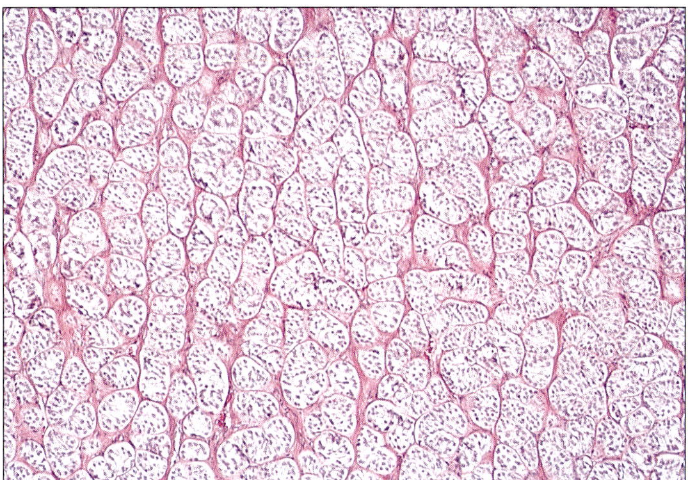

Figure 6.15 Sertoli cell adenoma in testis of androgen insensitivity syndrome. The tumor is composed of closely packed tubules filled with Sertoli cells.

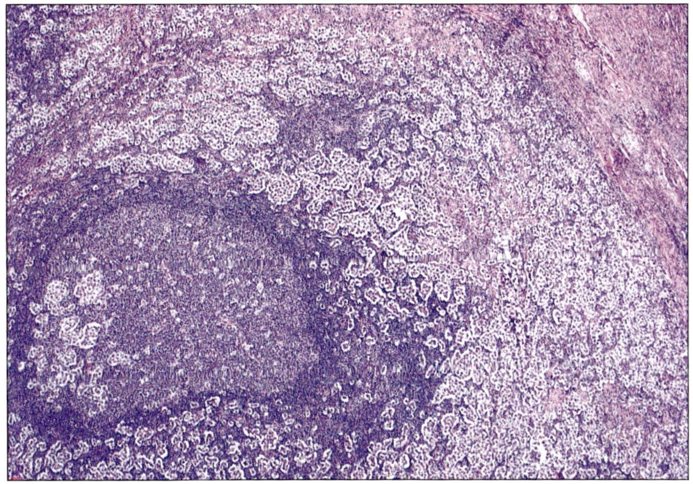

Figure 6.16 Seminoma in testis of androgen insensitivity syndrome. The tumor contains a large lymphoid follicle.

References

1. Scully RE. Neoplasia associated with anomalous sexual development and abnormal sex chromosomes. *Pediatr Adolesc Endrocrinol* 8:203–217, 1981.
2. Rutgers JL, Scully RE. Pathology of the testis in intersex syndromes. *Semin Diagn Pathol* 4:275–291, 1987.
3. Robboy SJ, Miller T, Donahue PK, et al. Dysgenesis of testicular and streak gonads in the syndrome of mixed gonadal dysgenesis. *Hum Pathol* 13:700–716, 1982.
4. Müller J, Skakkebaek NE, Ritzen, M, et al. Carcinoma in situ of the testis in children with 45,X/46,XY gonadal dysgenesis. *J Pediatr* 106:431–436, 1985.
5. Scully RE. Gonadoblastoma: A review of 74 cases. *Cancer* 25:1340–1356, 1970.
6. Ishida T, Tagatz GE, Okagaki T. Gonadoblastoma: Ultrastructural evidence for testicular origin. *Cancer* 37:1770–1781, 1976.
7. Manuel M, Katayama KP, Jones HW. The age of occurrence of gonadal tumors in intersex patients with a Y chromosome. *Am J Obstet Gynecol* 124:293–300, 1976.
8. Talerman A. The pathology of gonadal neoplasms composed of germ cells and sex cord stroma derivatives. *Pathol Res Pract* 170:24–38, 1980.
9. Bolen JW. Mixed germ cell-sex cord stroma tumor: A gonadal tumor distinct from gonadoblastoma. *Am J Clin Pathol* 75:565–573, 1981.
10. Young RH, Lawrence WD, Scully RE. Juvenile granulosa cell tumor: Another neoplasm associated with abnormal chromosomes and ambiguous genitalia: A report of three cases. *Am J Surg Pathol* 9:737–743, 1985.
11. Van Niekerk WA. True hermaphroditism. *Pediatr Adolesc Endocrinol* 8:80–99, 1981.
12. O'Dowd J, Gaffney EF, Young RH. Malignant sex cord–stromal tumor in a patient with the androgen insensitivity syndrome. *Histopathology*, in press.
13. Müller J. Morphometry and histology of gonads from twelve children and adolescents with the androgen insensitivity (testicular feminization) syndrome. *J Clin Endocrinol Metabol* 59:785–789, 1984.
14. Grünberger W. Cited by Müller J. Abnormal infantile germ cells and development of carcinoma-in-situ in maldeveloped testes. Boston, Blackwell Scientific Publications, 1987, 26 pp.

7 Hematopoietic and Metastatic Tumors

Malignant Lymphoma

Malignant lymphomas account for approximately 5% of all testicular neoplasms and approximately 50% of testicular tumors in men over 60 years of age.[1,2] Lymphoma is the most common tumor that involves both testes, with the frequency of bilaterality ranging up to 38%.[2–5] Involvement of the second testis is much more often metachronous than synchronous. In most cases, testicular lymphoma is a local manifestation of more widespread disease that is evident synchronously or within a short interval after treatment of the testicular tumor. Occasional patients with tumor confined to the testis are apparently cured by appropriate treatment.

Gross examination of a testis involved by lymphoma reveals partial or complete replacement by a fleshy or firm homogeneous mass, which may be cream-colored (Figure 7.1), tan, pale yellow, or slightly pink; lobulation is occasionally conspicuous; areas of necrosis may be present. This gross appearance closely resembles that of a typical or spermatocytic seminoma, but lymphoma involves the epididymis (Figure 7.1) or spermatic cord much more often than either form of seminoma. For example, in one representative series,[5] epididymal involvement by lymphoma was present on gross inspection in one half of the cases. Similar spread is seen in only 8% of seminomas.[6]

Low-power microscopic examination often suggests the diagnosis of lymphoma because of the predominant intertubular infiltration of the neoplastic cells (Figure 7.2), a finding that is not conspicuous in most other types of testicular neoplasia. Lymphoma cells also invade and fill tubules in approximately one third of the cases (Figure 7.3), but the involved tubules almost invariably lie within the tumor, in contrast to the tubular involvement outside the tumor that occurs in most cases of seminoma. Staining for reticulum fibrils in cases of lymphoma reveals separation of the fibrils in the walls of the tubules that have been invaded (Figure 7.4), in contrast to condensation of the fibrils in the walls of tubules invaded by seminoma cells. In some cases, extensive sclerosis is present (Figure 7.5). Microscopic evidence of extratesticular spread is common. Most testicular lymphomas are of the diffuse, large cell type,[7–9] although other types may be encountered. Burkitt's lymphoma is particularly common in some regions of the world. Hodgkin's disease of the testis is extremely rare.

Testicular lymphomas must be distinguished from other neoplasms, specifically typical seminoma, spermatocytic seminoma, embryonal carcinoma, and nonneoplastic inflammatory processes such as viral orchitis and granulomatous orchitis. Although the characteristic pattern of growth of lymphoma is helpful in the differential diagnosis, reliable distinction depends on appreciation of the morphologic features and staining characteristics of the neoplastic cells. Seminoma cells, unlike lymphoma cells, have prominent cell membranes, abundant glycogen-rich cytoplasm, and rounded but focally flattened central nuclei with one or a few prominent nucleoli. The cells of spermatocytic seminomas have mostly spherical, dark nuclei of unequal size and glycogen-free cytoplasm, and those of embryonal carcinoma are anaplastic, sometimes contain clear cytoplasm, and grow in a variety of distinctive epithelial patterns. Embryonal carcinoma cells are also positive immunohistochemically for cytokeratins, whereas lymphomas are negative for these antigens and typically positive for leukocyte common antigen.

The gross and histologic appearances of viral orchitis and granulomatous orchitis may be confused with those of lymphoma, but the heterogeneous and benign-appearing inflammatory cellular infiltrates of these lesions contrast with the homogeneous and malignant-appearing infiltrates of lymphoma. Also, viral orchitis has a patchy instead of a diffuse distribution.

Multiple Myeloma and Plasmacytoma

Testicular involvement occurs in approximately 2% of patients with multiple myeloma, but in such cases, the tumor is usually not detected until autopsy. Very rarely, the involvement is clinically evident and in a few cases testicular enlargement precedes recognition of the existence of the disease. Cases of solitary plasmacytoma of the testis and testicular plasmacytoma associated with similar tumors of other organs have also been reported.[10,11] The gross features (Figure 7.6) and microscopic patterns of testicular involvement by myeloma and plasmacytoma are essentially similar to those of malignant lymphomas.

Leukemia

Microscopic involvement of the testis has been found at autopsy in 64% of patients with acute leukemia, and 22% of those with chronic leukemia.[12] The testis is enlarged in 5% to 10% of the cases at autopsy. Testicular swelling is evident during life in only 5% of patients with leukemia, and testicular enlargement as the presenting manifestation of the disease is exceptionally rare. Testicular leukemic involvement is now seen most commonly by the pathologist in biopsy specimens from live patients obtained to detect relapse after treatment of acute lymphoblastic leukemia (Figure 7.7). The testis may serve as a sanctuary for the neoplastic cells in such patients. On microscopic examination the pattern of leukemic infiltration is similar to that of lymphoma (Figure 7.7), with tubular invasion in some of the cases.

Metastatic Tumors

If one excludes lymphomas and leukemias from the category of secondary tumors, carcinomas of the prostate gland (Figures 7.8, 7.9) and lung are the tumors that most commonly metastasize to the testis, with the former accounting for approximately one third and the latter approximately one fifth of the cases reported in the literature. The next most frequent sources of testicular metastasis have been malignant melanoma of the skin (Figures 7.10, 7.11) and carcinomas of the colon, kidney, stomach, and pancreas.[13–15] Occasional carcinoid tumors metastatic to the testis have also been reported.[16] Testicular metastases account for a significant proportion of testicular neoplasms in men over 50 years of age. They usually occur in patients with a known primary tumor elsewhere, but a testicular mass has been the presenting manifestation in almost 10% of the cases. The primary tumor in these cases has been in the prostate gland (three cases), kidney (two cases), pancreas (one case), stomach (one case), colon (one case), and liver (one case).[15,17] In one case, the tumor was a carcinoid, which was probably of gastrointestinal origin, and in another case, the primary site was never determined. Testicular metastases are bilateral in 15% of the cases.

Gross examination usually reveals single or multiple nodules but diffuse involvement is occasionally seen. The presence of multiple nodules should raise the possibility of metastasis, particularly in a patient over 50 years of age. A microscopic feature suggestive of metastasis is a predominant localization of the tumor in the interstitium (Figures 7.8, 7.10). Metastatic tumors, however, may also invade and fill the tubules. The distinctive microscopic features of most metastases in routinely stained sections are usually incompatible with a primary testicular tumor. In occasional difficult cases, special stains, particularly for mucin, argyrophil granules and melanin, and immunoperoxidase studies, particularly for prostatic carcinoma (Figure 7.9) and malignant melanoma (Figure 7.11), may be helpful in establishing or confirming the diagnosis.

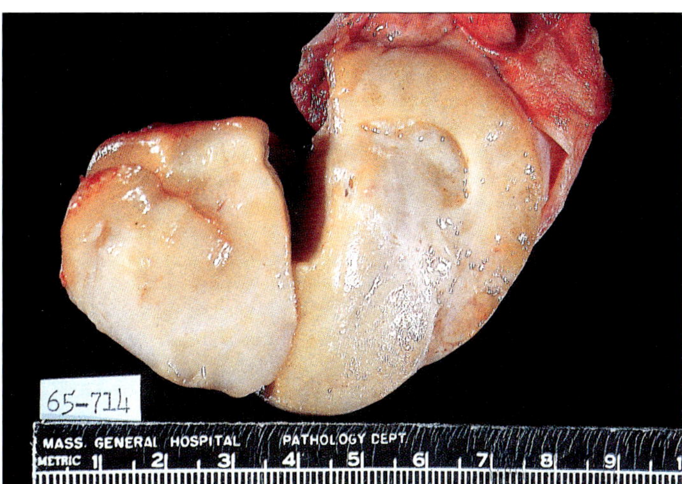

Figure 7.1 Lymphoma. The testis and epididymis are totally replaced by cream-colored to pale yellow neoplastic tissue.

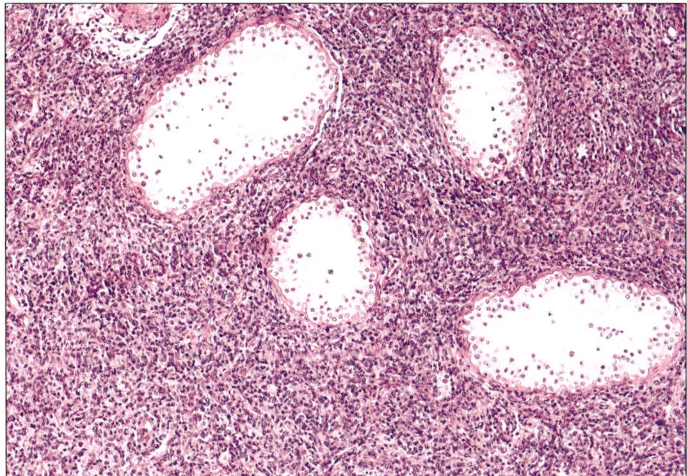

Figure 7.2 Lymphoma. The testicular tubules are widely separated by an infiltrate of uniform neoplastic cells.

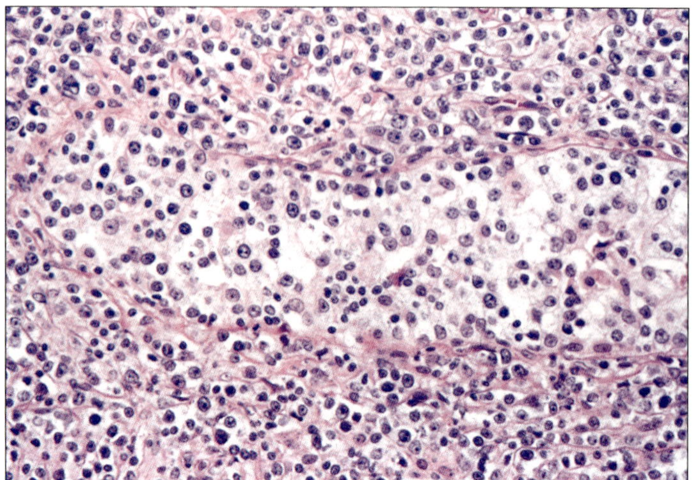

Figure 7.3 Lymphoma. A tubule has been extensively invaded by lymphoma cells.

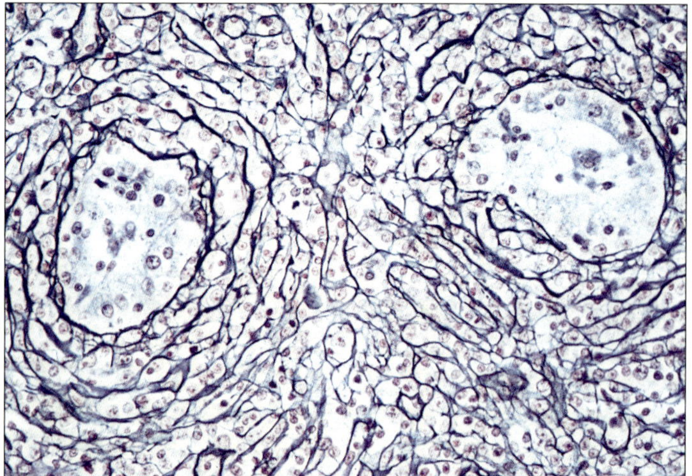

Figure 7.4 Lymphoma. Staining for reticulum reveals separation of the fibrils in the walls of the tubules by the infiltrating neoplastic cells.

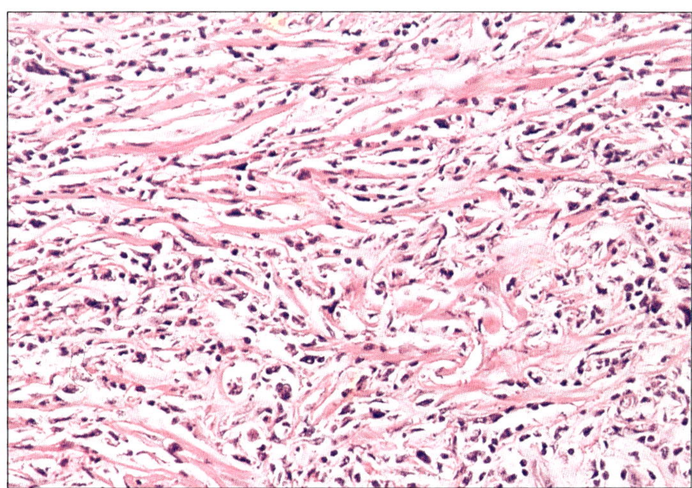

Figure 7.5 Lymphoma. This tumor has undergone extensive sclerosis.

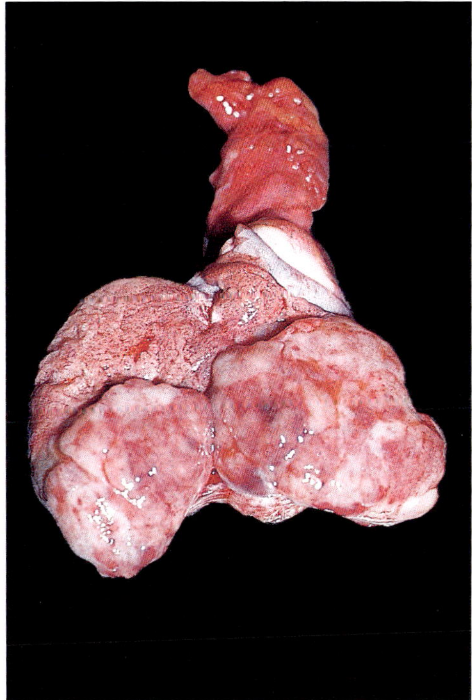

Figure 7.6 Plasmacytoma. This patient also had a plasmacytoma of the nasopharynx and the contralateral epididymis.

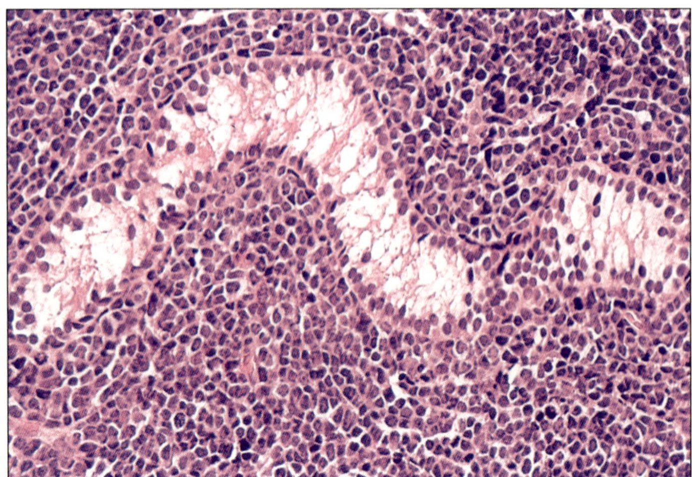

Figure 7.7 Acute lymphoblastic leukemia. An immature testicular tubule is surrounded by uniform, immature neoplastic cells.

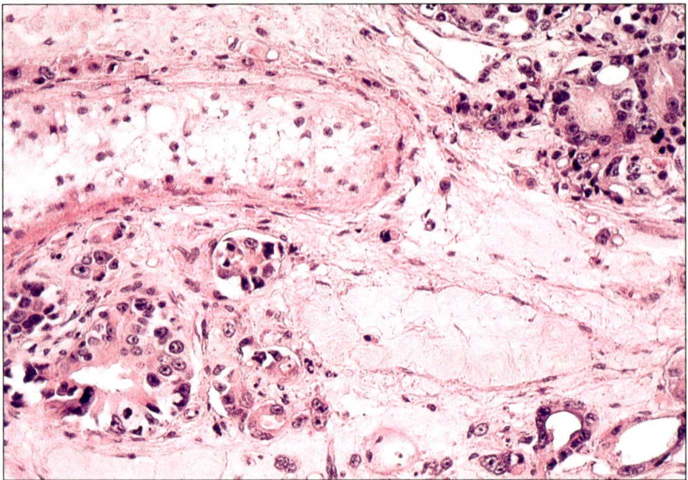

Figure 7.8 Metastatic adenocarcinoma of the prostate. Numerous neoplastic acini are present in the interstitial tissue.

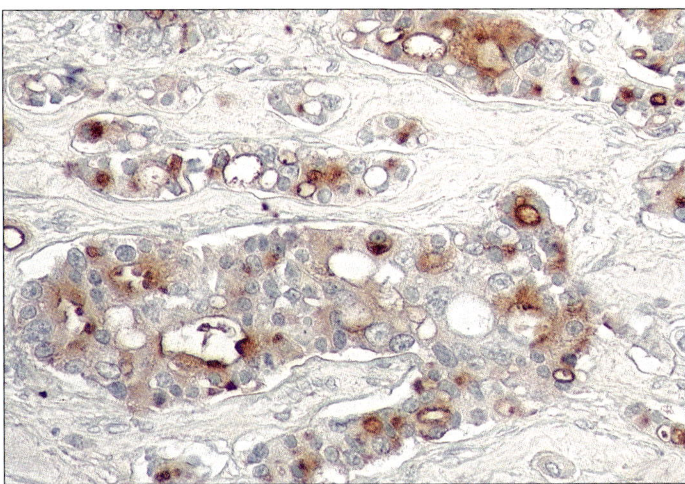

Figure 7.9 Metastatic adenocarcinoma of the prostate. The tumor cells illustrated in the previous figure are stained immunohistochemically for prostate-specific antigen.

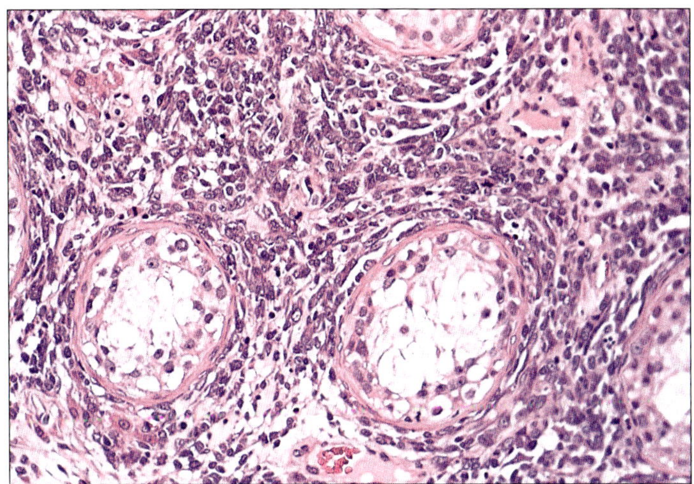

Figure 7.10 Metastatic malignant melanoma. The tubules are separated by a diffuse proliferation of neoplastic cells.

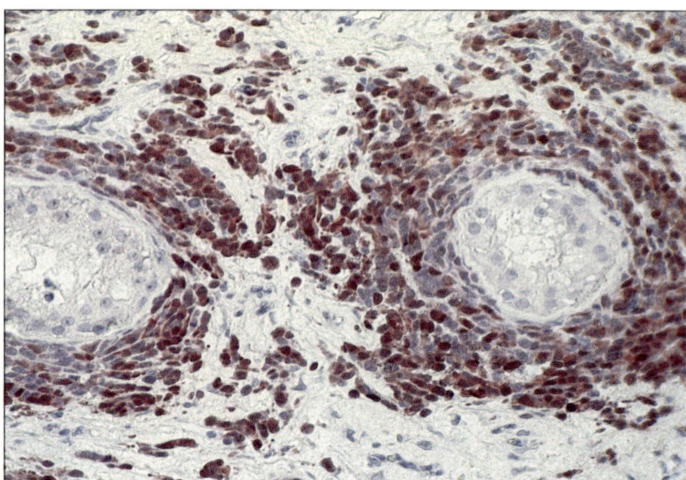

Figure 7.11 Metastatic malignant melanoma. The tumor illustrated in the previous figure is stained immunohistochemically for S-100 protein.

References

1. Abell MR, Holtz F. Testicular and paratesticular neoplasms in patients 60 years of age and older. *Cancer* 21:852–870, 1968.
2. Gowing NFC. Malignant lymphoma of the testis. *Br J Urol* 36:85–94, 1964.
3. Kiely JM, Massey BD, Harrison EG, Utz DC. Lymphoma of the testis. *Cancer* 26:847–852, 1970.
4. Sussman EB, Hajdu SI, Lieberman PH, Whitmore WF. Malignant lymphoma of the testis: A clinicopathological study of 37 cases. *J Urol* 118:1004–1007, 1977.
5. Talerman A. Primary malignant lymphoma of the testis. *J Urol* 118:783–786, 1977.
6. Mostofi FK, Price EB Jr. *Atlas of Tumor Pathology,* 2nd series, Fascicle 8. *Tumors of the Male Genital System*. Washington, DC, Armed Forces Institute of Pathology, 1973.
7. Paladugu RR, Bearman RM, Rappaport H. Malignant lymphoma with primary manifestation in the gonad: A clinicopathologic study of 38 patients. *Cancer* 45:561–571, 1980.
8. Duncan PR, Checa F, Gowing NFC, et al. Extranodal non-Hodgkin's lymphoma presenting in the testicle: A clinical and pathologic study of 24 cases. *Cancer* 45:1578–1584, 1980.
9. Turner RR, Colby TV, MacKintosh FR. Testicular lymphomas: A clinicopathologic study of 35 cases. *Cancer* 48:2095–2102, 1981.
10. Levin HS, Mostofi FK. Symptomatic plasmacytoma of the testis. *Cancer* 25:1193–1203, 1970.
11. Young RH, Scully RE. Miscellaneous neoplasms and non-neoplastic lesions. In: *Pathology of the Testis*, Talerman A, Roth LM, eds. *Contemporary Issues in Surgical Pathology,* vol 7. New York, Churchill Livingstone, 1986, chap 5.
12. Givler RL. Testicular involvement in leukemia and lymphoma. *Cancer* 23:1290–1295, 1969.
13. Price EB, Mostofi FK. Secondary carcinoma of the testis. *Cancer* 10:592–595, 1957.
14. Tiltman AJ. Metastatic tumors in the testis. *Histopathology* 3:31–37, 1979.
15. Haupt HM, Mann RB, Trump DL, Abeloff MD. Metastatic carcinoma involving the testis: Clinical and pathologic distinction from primary testicular neoplasms. *Cancer* 54:709–714, 1984.
16. Berdjis CC, Mostofi FK. Carcinoid tumors of the testis. *J Urol* 118:777–782, 1977.
17. Young RH, Van Patter HT, Scully RE. Hepatocellular carcinoma metastatic to the testis. *Am J Clin Pathol* 87:117–120, 1987.

Miscellaneous Tumors Including Adnexal Tumors

8

Adenomatoid Tumor

The adenomatoid tumor is a benign tumor of mesothelial origin that is located most often in the epididymis (Figure 8.1), usually at its lower pole, but it may also arise in or beneath the tunica albuginea of the testis (Figure 8.2) or in the spermatic cord.[1,2] Occasionally, the testicular parenchyma is involved by local extension.[3,4] This tumor is the most common benign neoplasm of the testicular adnexa, accounting for 60% of the cases in a recent study.[5] The adenomatoid tumor has been reported in all age groups. It is almost always unilateral and solitary and rarely exceeds 5 cm in diameter. Although typically round or oval and well demarcated, it may be plaquelike and it may have an ill-defined margin. It is composed of solid, tan to gray-white, glistening tissue (Figure 8.1); when it involves the testis prominently, it may resemble a germ cell tumor, especially a seminoma.

Microscopic examination reveals in varying proportions tubules, which are round, oval or slitlike and range from very small to cystic, small cords and clusters of cells, and individual cells containing large intracytoplasmic vacuoles (Figures 8.3 to 8.6). The neoplastic cells lining the tubules vary from flat to columnar and contain moderate to large amounts of dense or vacuolated cytoplasm (Figure 8.6). The stroma, which is often prominent, is usually fibrous and sometimes hyalinized; it may contain smooth muscle, which rarely predominates, and lymphoid aggregates may be prominent (Figure 8.3). The infiltrative borders of some adenomatoid tumors may suggest malignancy (Figure 8.4), and rare examples have disquieting cytological features as well.

Adenomatoid tumors are most apt to be confused with malignant mesotheliomas. Knowledge of the gross characteristics of the mass is important in avoiding this potentially serious error. Malignant mesotheliomas are typically large, diffuse tumors, in contrast to adenomatoid tumors. Certain microscopic patterns of mesothelioma, such as papillary and biphasic, are also incompatible with the diagnosis of an adenomatoid tumor and the degree of atypia in almost all mesotheliomas exceeds that acceptable for an adenomatoid tumor. The vacuolated cells and glandlike differentiation of the adenomatoid tumor rarely raise the question of a yolk sac tumor, but the typical high degree of differentiation of the former and its failure to stain for AFP facilitate the differential diagnosis.

Malignant Mesothelioma

Malignant mesotheliomas of the tunica vaginalis, 24 cases of which have been reported, are often associated with a hydrocele, which may recur repeatedly after tapping[6,7]; a mass or ill-defined firmness may be palpated but the diagnosis of a neoplasm is often not apparent until exploration has been performed. A history of asbestos exposure has been elicited in one fourth of the reported cases.[7]

Gross examination reveals tumor tissue coating the tunica vaginalis to varying extents (Figure 8.7) or multiple nodules on its surface. Microscopic examination reveals papillary, tubular, diffuse, and, less commonly, biphasic or fibrous patterns similar to those encountered in malignant mesotheliomas of the pleura and peritoneal cavity (Figures 8.8 to 8.11). The neoplastic cells are typically cuboidal, with moderate amounts of eosinophilic cytoplasm in well-differentiated tumors, but may have highly malignant features in other cases.

Tumors of Ovarian Epithelial Types

Rare testicular or paratesticular tumors have microscopic features similar to those of ovarian tumors of the surface epithelial type.[8–11] These neoplasms have included seven serous tumors of borderline malignancy (Figures 8.12, 8.13), one serous carcinoma, one well-differentiated endometrioid adenocarcinoma with squamous differentiation, one mucinous cystadenoma, one mucinous cystadenocarcinoma, one clear cell adenocarcinoma (Figures 8.14, 8.15), four Brenner tumors, and one benign tumor of mixed cell types. These tumors occurred in patients from 14 to 68 years of age (average, 44 years). The exact location of the tumor was known for 15 cases. Seven primarily or entirely involved the testicular parenchyma; four, the tunica vaginalis; and four, paratesticular tissue. In one case, two separate intratesticular tumors were present,[11] and in another, multiple nodules studded the tunica vaginalis.[9] Only the clear cell adenocarcinoma is known to have been clinically malignant. One serous borderline tumor[11] was immunoreactive for OC-125 and had ultrastructural features suggestive of a müllerian nature.

The microscopic appearance of these tumors is so distinctive that their correct diagnosis is usually not difficult. Serous tumors may, however, be confused with carcinomas of the rete testis and mesotheliomas. The typical location of carcinomas of the rete testis in the hilus is helpful in the differential diagnosis. Although serous borderline tumors of the tunica vaginalis may be grossly indistinguishable from mesotheliomas, the papillae in well-differentiated mesotheliomas are lined by uniform cuboidal cells containing eosinophilic cytoplasm; psammoma bodies are typically rare and cilia are absent.

One unique tumorlike lesion with a müllerian nature in the paratesticular region was a uteruslike structure composed of endometrial-type glands and stroma surrounded by bundles of smooth muscle (Figure 8.16). This lesion arose in an 82-year-old man who had received diethlystilbesterol for carcinoma of the prostate gland.[8]

Tumors of the Rete Testis

Four benign tumors of the rete testis designated adenoma, cystadenoma, and adenofibroma have been reported.[12,13] They were solid, cystic, or both on gross examination. Microscopic examination showed continuity with the rete testis and cystic and papillary patterns, with the cysts and papillae lined by benign-appearing epithelium (Figure 8.17). Rete carcinomas typically occur in men over 50 years of age; approximately one fourth of them are associated with a hydrocele.[14,15] They are usually solid, but may contain cysts. Microscopic examination reveals tubular, papillary, and solid patterns (Figures 8.18, 8.19). The tubules are typically elongated, compressed, and slitlike. The papillae, which may project into cysts, may be small and cellular or large with fibrous or hyalinized cores. The stroma is often prominent and may be extensively hyalinized. The neoplastic cells are typically small and cuboidal with scanty cytoplasm; nuclear stratification and at least moderate nuclear pleomorphism and mitotic activity are usually present.

Metastatic adenocarcinomas, particularly from the lung, may simulate adenocarcinoma of the rete and a careful clinical investigation to exclude an extratesticular primary carcinoma is indicated before making a diagnosis. Support for the conclusion that a carcinoma arose in the rete is provided by a predominant location in the region of the rete and, of greater importance, the demonstration of a transition between the neoplastic cells and uninvolved rete epithelium. Rete adenocarcinomas should also be distinguished from serous tumors of the testis, as discussed above. One rete adenocarcinoma described in the literature had features suggestive of a serous tumor of borderline malignancy.[16] Mesotheliomas may also simulate rete carcinomas because, like the latter, they may have elongated, slitlike tubules. The distribution of the mesothelioma and the presence of other distinctive patterns, however, should help in the differential diagnosis. It should also be emphasized that in some atrophic testes a relatively prominent and seemingly hyperplastic rete may result in an erroneous suspicion of adenoma or carcinoma (Figure 8.20). Rarely, true hyperplasia of the rete testis occurs.[17,18]

Papillary Cystadenoma and Carcinoma of the Epididymis

Papillary cystadenomas of the epididymis occur over a wide age range and are bilateral in approximately one third of cases.[19] Approximately 17% of patients with von Hippel–Lindau disease have epididymal papillary cystadenomas, which may be the initial manifestation of the disease.[20] Most bilateral tumors of this type occur in patients with this syndrome. The diameter of the tumors has ranged up to 5 cm; they may be cystic, solid, or both. Microscopic examination discloses tubules and cysts, which may contain complex papillae lined by cytologically benign columnar cells (Figure 8.21). The lining cells often contain clear, glycogen-rich cytoplasm (Figure 8.22). We have seen one carcinoma of the epididymis, which was composed of clear cells and may have been the malignant counterpart of the papillary cystadenoma (Figure 8.23). Rare additional adenocarcinomas of the epididymis have been reported,[21] but the diagnosis should be made with caution and only after metastasis has been carefully excluded. It should be remembered that the epithelium of the normal epididymis often shows a cribriform pattern and occasionally contains atypical cells (Figure 8.24) similar to those seen more commonly in the seminal vesicle.[22]

Retinal Anlage Tumor

Nine examples of this rare tumor, which has also been designated melanotic neuroectodermal tumor, melanotic hamartoma, and melanotic progonoma, have been reported in the epididymis.[23–25] Eight of the nine patients were 10 months of age or less, and one was 2 years old. Eight tumors were 4 cm or less in diameter; one replaced the epididymis.[23] Most of the tumors were well circumscribed and round to oval. The sectioned surfaces are typically brown or black, at least focally, but may be predominantly cream-colored or gray (Figure 8.25). Microscopic examination reveals sheets, nests (Figure 8.26), cords, and spaces composed of or lined by cells of two types (Figures 8.27, 8.28); large cuboidal cells, many of which contain melanin pigment in their cytoplasm (Figure 8.28); and smaller cells with round to oval, hyperchromatic nuclei and scanty cytoplasm, resembling the cells of a neuroblastoma (Figure 8.27). The latter cells predominate and may exhibit considerable mitotic activity (Figure 8.27). The tumor cells sometimes lie in a fibrous stroma. Because of the cellularity, mitotic activity, and predominant component of small cells, the appearance of this tumor usually brings into the differential diagnosis other small cell malignant tumors that occur in this location in children, particularly a paratesticular rhabdomyosarcoma. Other diagnoses such as malignant lymphoma are occasionally suggested. Careful scrutiny to identify melanin in small cell tumors occurring in this location in children is crucial in establishing the correct diagnosis. Masson-Fontana staining may aid in the identification of the pigment (Figure 8.29). Despite their relatively ominous appearance, only one tumor of this type has been reported to be clinically malignant. It occurred in a 5-month-old boy, exhibited lymphatic invasion, and was associated with microscopic foci of metastatic tumor in inguinal and retroperitoneal lymph nodes at the time of exploration.[23] Although the child did not receive adjuvant therapy, follow-up examination over a period of four years was uneventful.

Soft Tissue Tumors

Benign and malignant soft tissue tumors are very rare in the testis but are relatively common in the spermatic cord and epididymis (Figure 8.30). After the adenomatoid tumor, the leiomyoma is the most common benign tumor at this location.[5] Occasional hemangiomas of the testis (Figure 8.31),[26] and sporadic examples of fibroma (Figure 8.32), lipoma, and neurofibroma have been reported.[27] Most of the reported malignant tumors of soft tissue type occurring in and adjacent to the testis have been rhabdomyosarcomas in children. They are typically paratesticular,[28,29] although involvement of the testicular parenchyma does occur.[28] Rare rhabdomyosarcomas originating within the testis in adults have also been described.[30,31] A low-grade leiomyosarcoma that arose in the testis of a 55-year-old man has also been reported,[32] as has an osteosarcoma in the testis of a 63-year-old man.[33] In a recent large study of paratesticular tumors,[5] the 34 sarcomas comprised 14 rhabdomyosarcomas, nine liposarcomas, seven leiomyosarcomas, and four malignant fibrous histiocytomas. The diagnosis of a pure sarcoma of any type in the testis (Figure 8.33) should only be made after thorough sampling has been performed to identify an underlying tumor from which the sarcoma may have arisen, such as a teratoma or spermatocytic seminoma. Additionally, as unclassified sex cord–stromal tumors may have a predominantly malignant-appearing mesenchymal component, the diagnosis of pure sarcoma of the testis should be made only after extensive sampling has excluded minor foci of epithelial differentiation, which might place the tumor in the sex cord–stromal category.

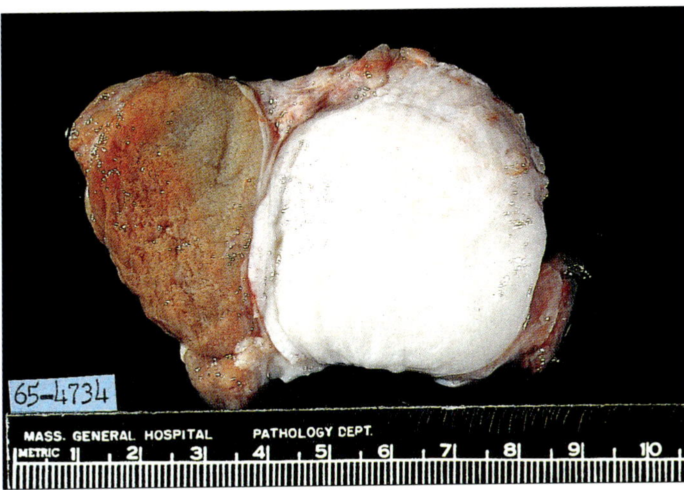

Figure 8.1 Adenomatoid tumor of the epididymis. The neoplastic tissue is cream-colored and bulging.

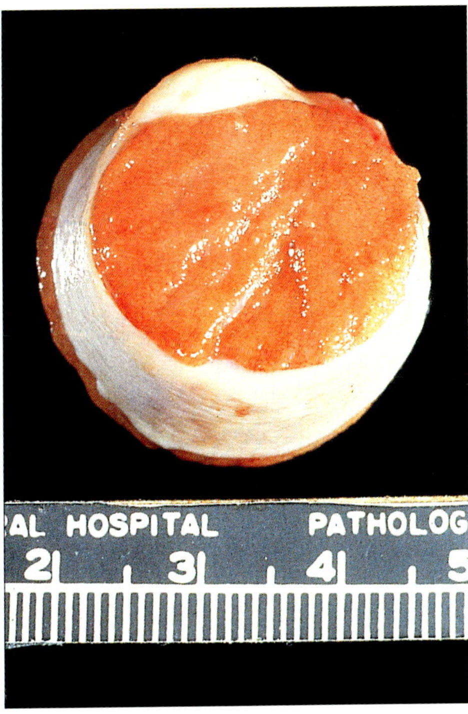

Figure 8.2 Adenomatoid tumor in the upper portion of the tunica albuginea.

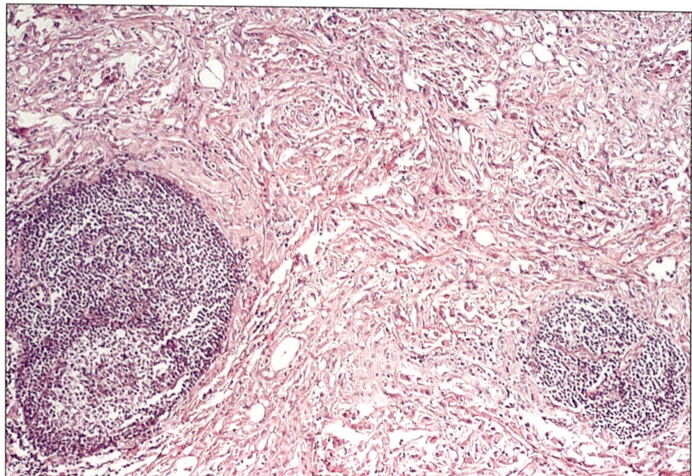

Figure 8.3 Adenomatoid tumor of the epididymis. The tumor is characterized by small glandlike structures and vacuoles in a dense fibrous stroma containing lymphoid aggregates.

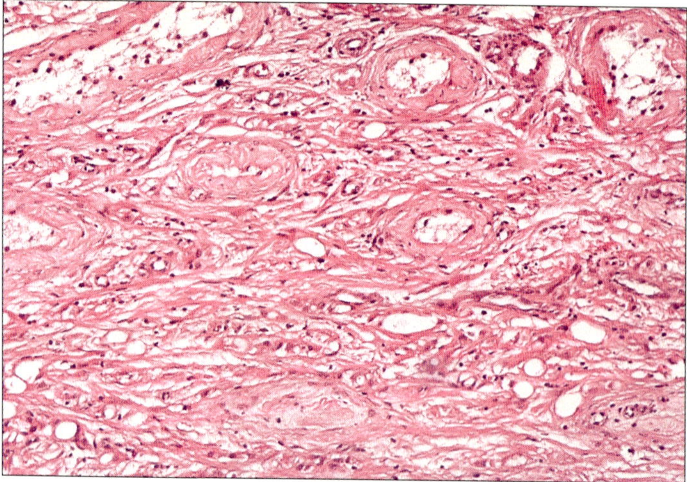

Figure 8.4 Adenomatoid tumor. The tumor is composed of small acini and vacuoles in a dense fibrous stroma, and infiltrates the testis.

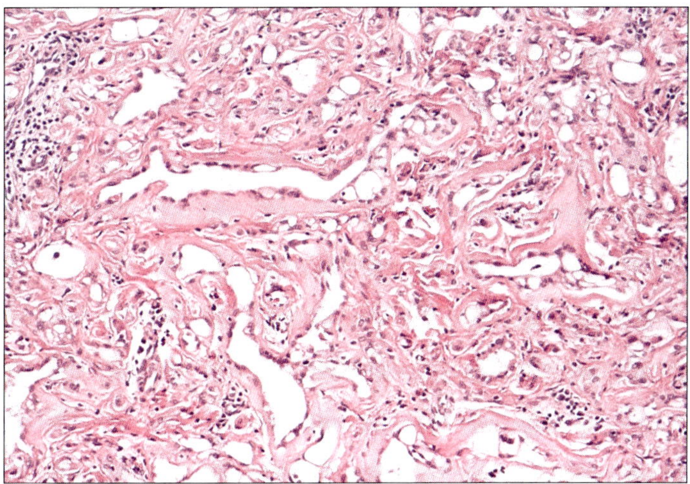

Figure 8.5 Adenomatoid tumor of the epididymis. The tumor is made up of glandlike structures, tubules, and vacuoles in a dense fibrous stroma.

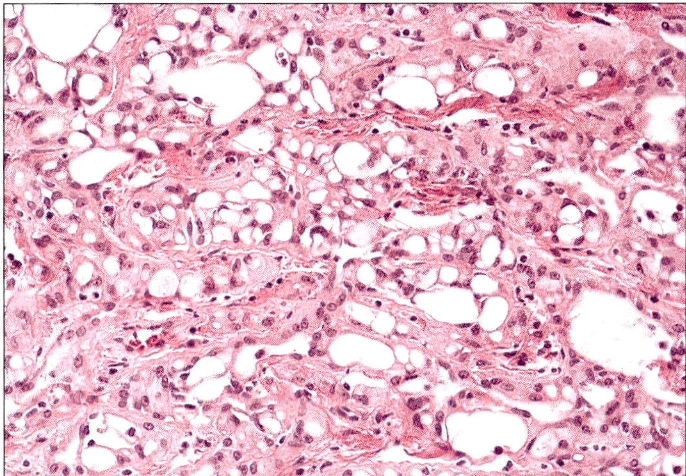

Figure 8.6 Adenomatoid tumor of the epididymis. The tumor is composed of tubular structures containing vacuolated cells, glandlike structures, and vacuoles in a fibrous stroma.

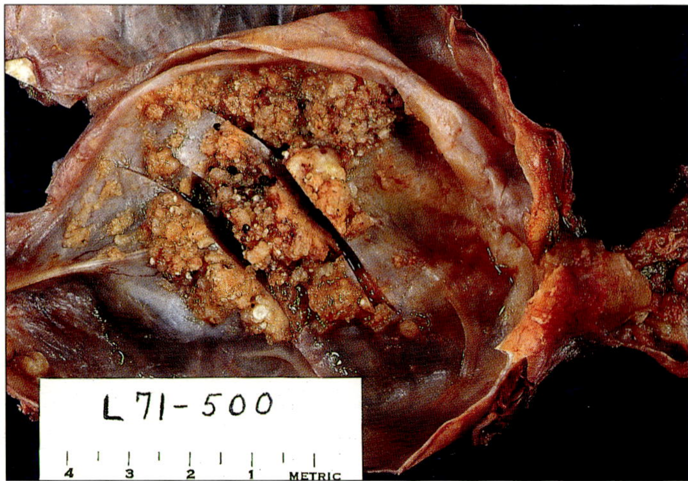

Figure 8.7 Mesothelioma of the tunica vaginalis. The tunica vaginalis is extensively involved by confluent papillary neoplastic tissue.

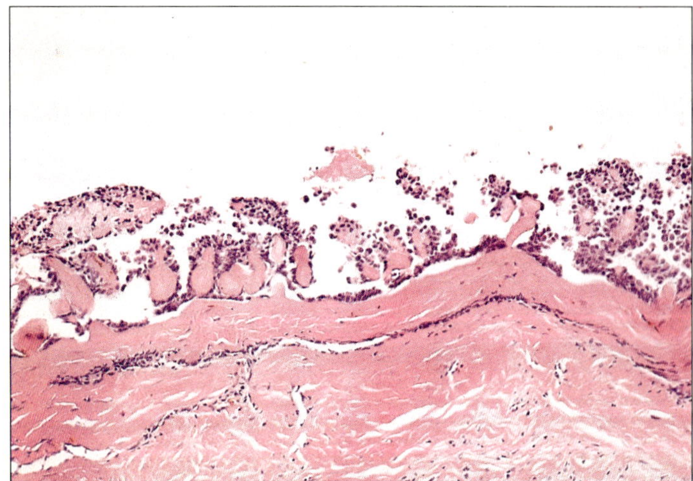

Figure 8.8 Mesothelioma of the tunica vaginalis. The tumor has a papillary pattern and is growing on the surface of the thickened, hyalinized tunica vaginalis.

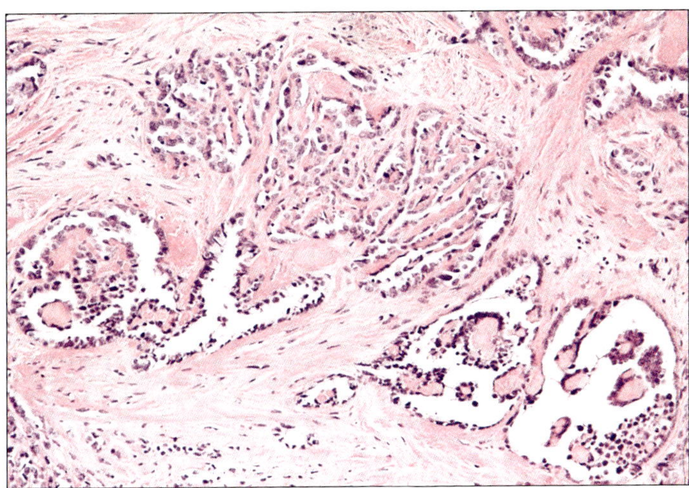

Figure 8.9 Mesothelioma of the tunica vaginalis. The tumor has tubular and papillary patterns.

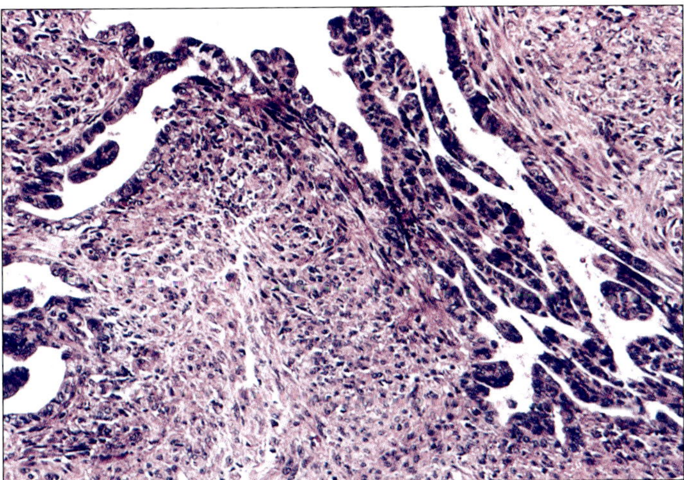

Figure 8.10 Mesothelioma of the tunica vaginalis. The tumor is poorly differentiated and has a biphasic pattern.

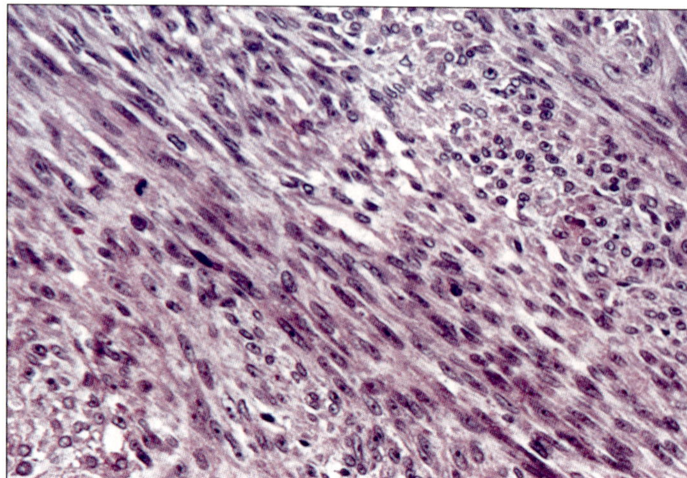

Figure 8.11 Mesothelioma of the tunica vaginalis. The sarcomatoid component of the tumor illustrated in the previous figure is characterized by intersecting fascicles of highly atypical spindle cells showing mitotic activity.

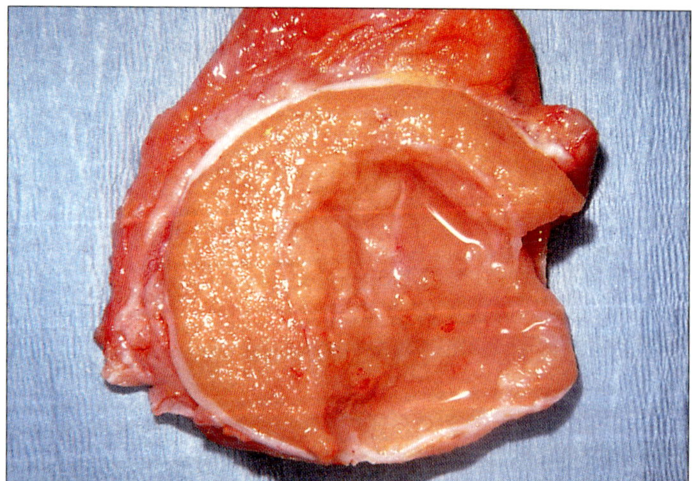

Figure 8.12 Serous papillary cystadenoma of borderline malignancy. The testis contains a cyst, with part of its lining covered by excrescences.

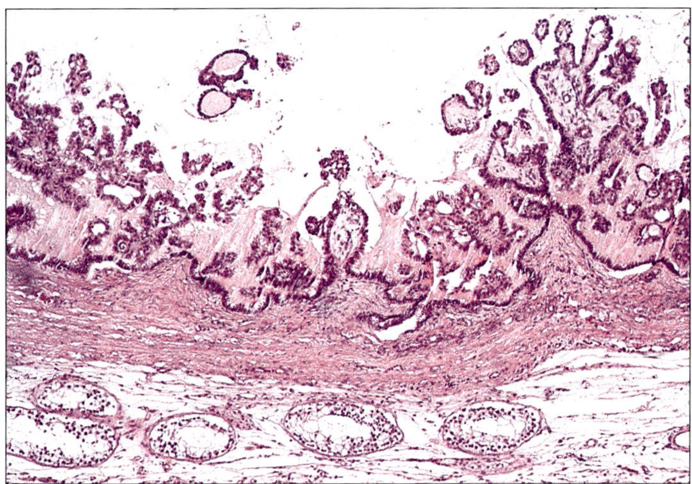

Figure 8.13 Serous papillary cystadenoma of borderline malignancy. The tumor is characterized by irregular papillae lined by stratified epithelium. There is cellular budding from the surfaces of the papillae. The cyst contains mucinous fluid.

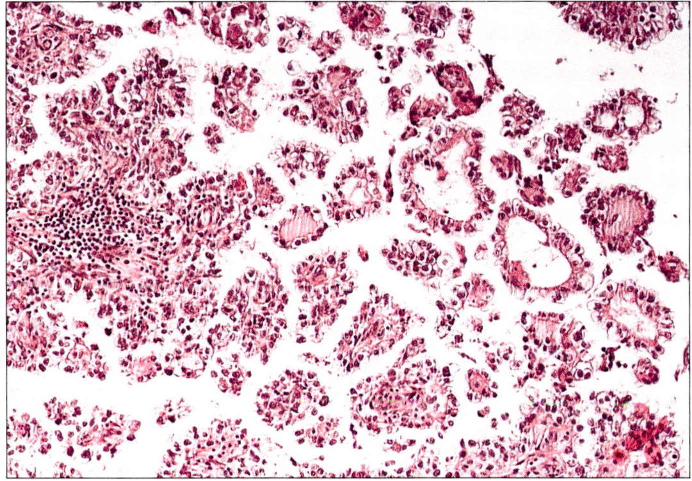

Figure 8.14 Clear cell papillary adenocarcinoma of the testis. This tumor replaced both the testis and epididymis.

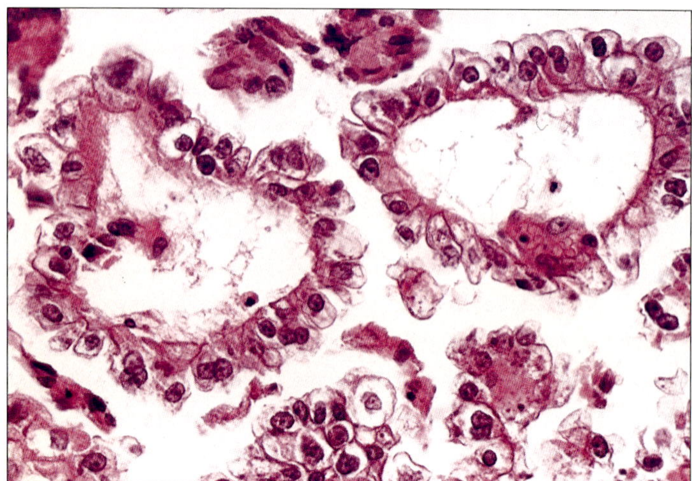

Figure 8.15 Clear cell papillary adenocarcinoma of the testis. The papillae are lined by large rounded cells containing abundant clear cytoplasm, which was stained for glycogen by the PAS technique.

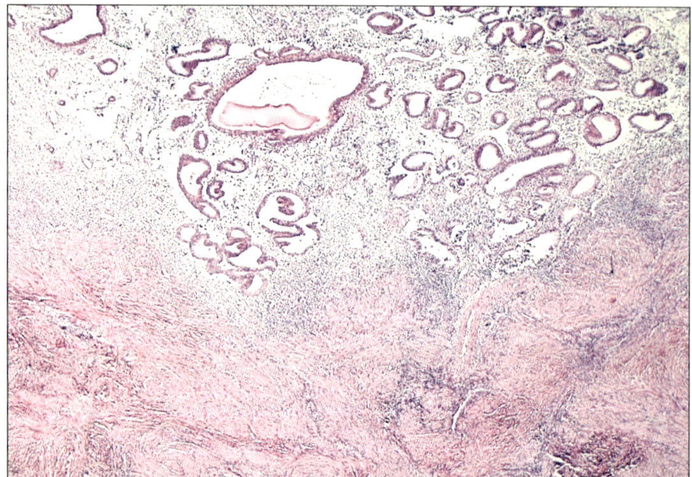

Figure 8.16 Endometriosis, paratesticular. This lesion was found in a patient receiving estrogen therapy for carcinoma of the prostate gland. The endometriotic tissue is bordered by hyperplastic smooth muscle.

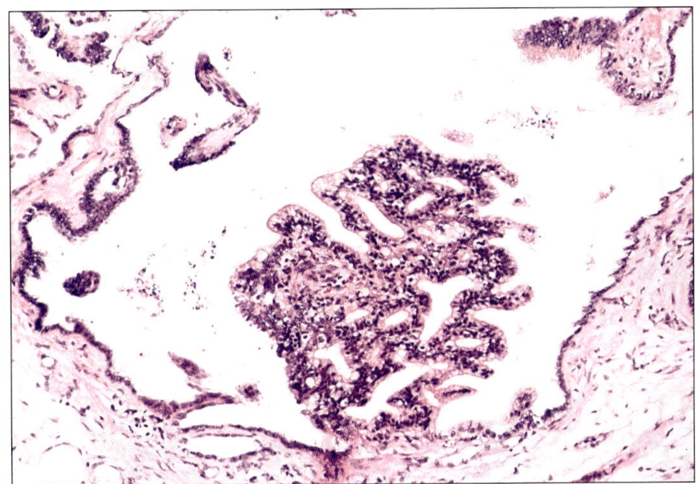

Figure 8.17 Papillary adenoma of the rete testis. The small papillary tumor lies in a dilated segment of the rete testis.

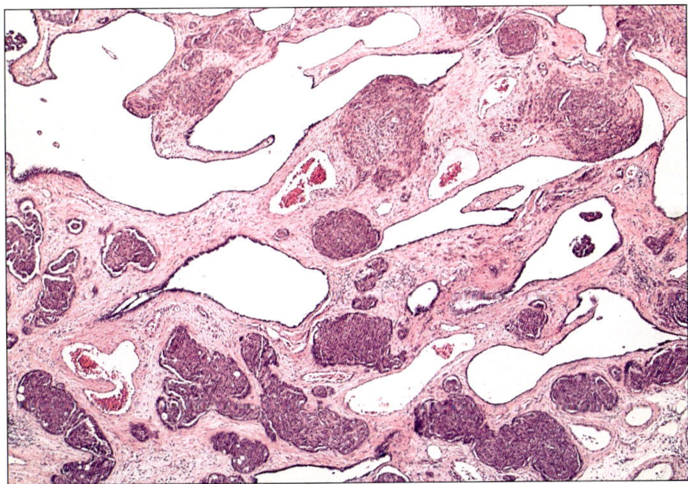

Figure 8.18 Carcinoma of the rete testis. Portions of the rete are occupied by papillary and solid masses of neoplastic epithelial cells. (Courtesy of Dr Lucien Nochomovitz.)

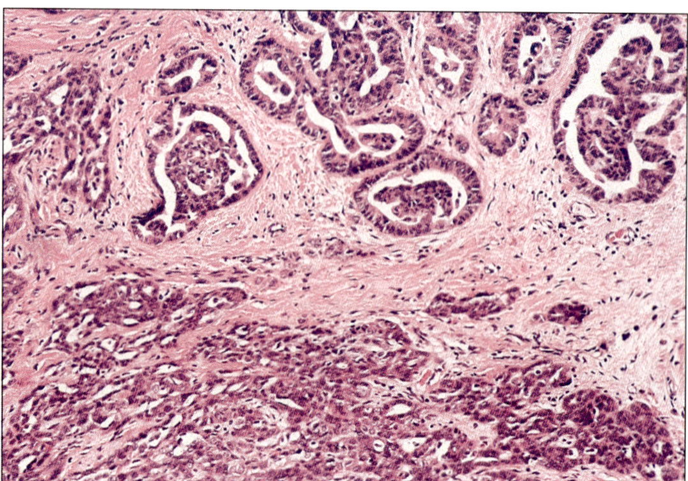

Figure 8.19 Carcinoma of the rete testis. The tumor has glandular and papillary patterns (above) and a retiform pattern (below). (Courtesy of Dr Lucien Nochomovitz.)

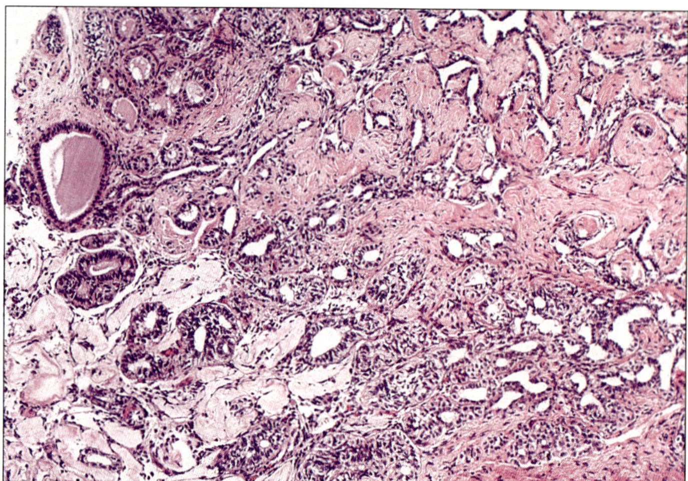

Figure 8.20 Pseudohyperplasia of the rete testis associated with testicular atrophy. The prominent rete lies in the right portion of the photomicrograph and atrophic, hyalinized testicular tubules are seen in the left portion. Straight tubules can be seen between the testicular tubules and the rete.

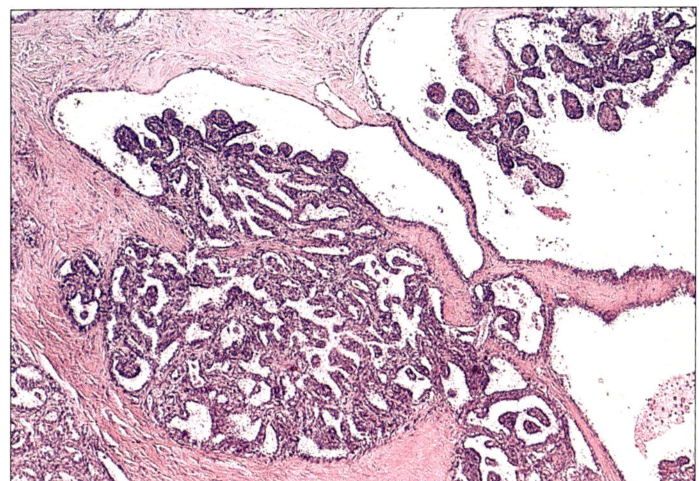

Figure 8.21 Papillary cystadenoma of the epididymis.

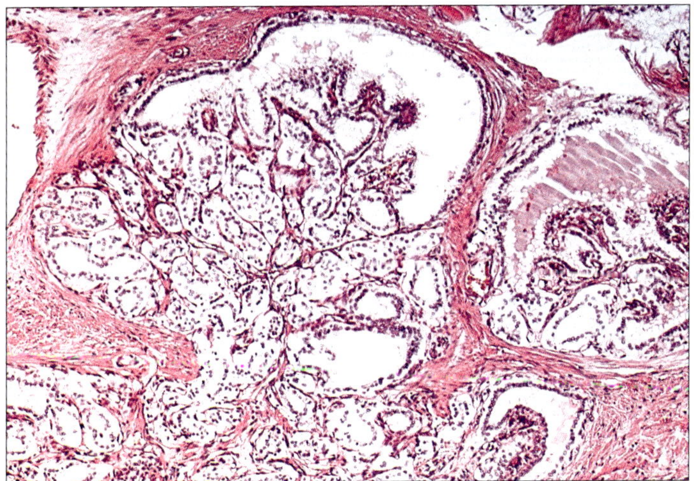

Figure 8.22 Papillary cystadenoma of the epididymis. This tumor was from a patient with von Hippel–Lindau's syndrome. The neoplastic cells contain abundant clear cytoplasm containing glycogen.

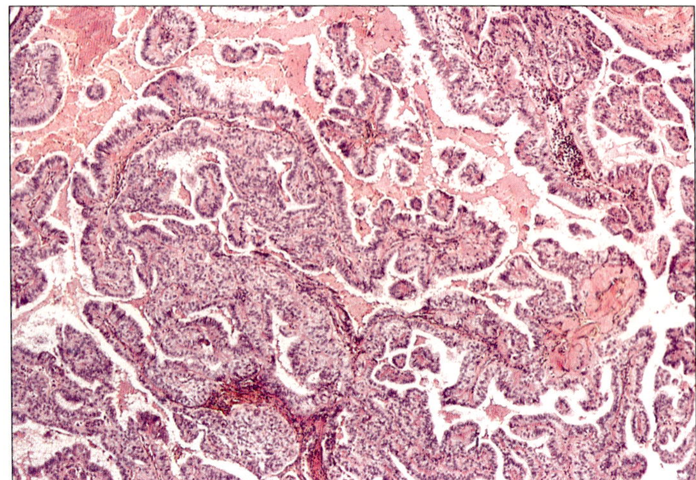

Figure 8.23 Papillary adenocarcinoma of the epididymis. This tumor metastasized to an inguinal lymph node.

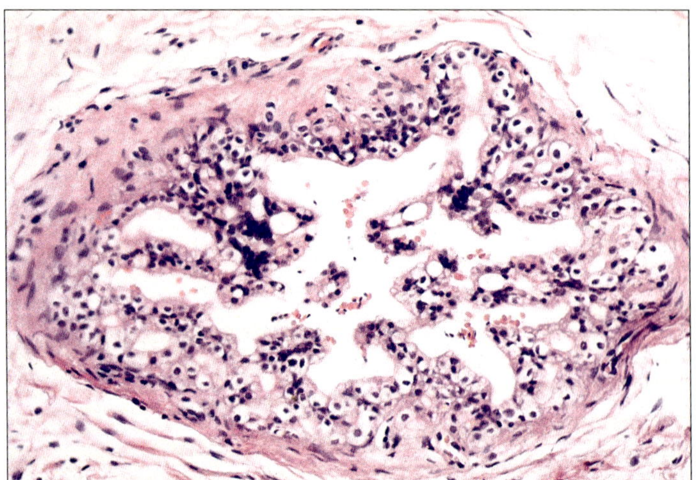

Figure 8.24 Atypical epithelial cells in the epididymis. The lining cells of this epididymal tubule are forming a few glandlike spaces. Some of the cells contain multiple smudgy nuclei.

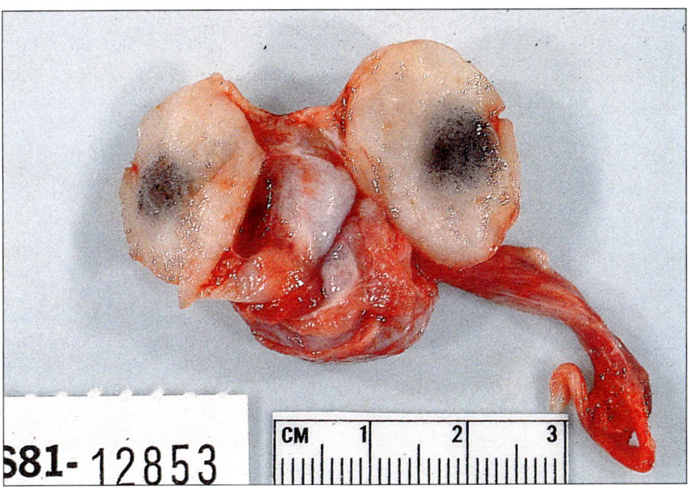

Figure 8.25 Retinal anlage tumor of the epididymis. Most of the tumor is composed of cream-colored tissue; a large central focus of melanin pigmentation is also visible. (Courtesy of Dr Bhagirath Majmudarr.)

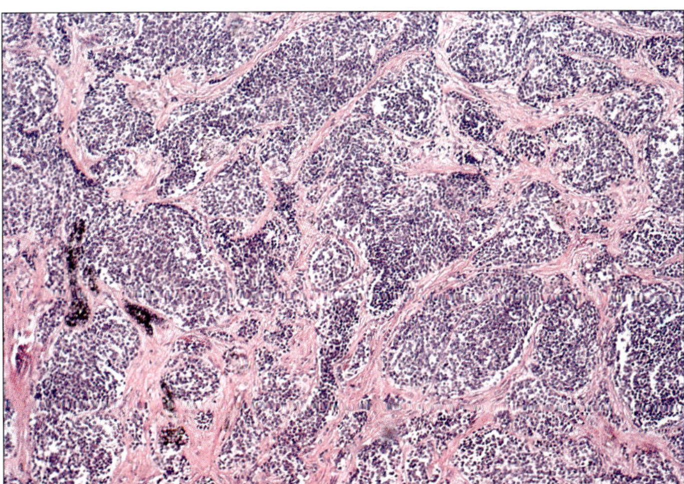

Figure 8.26 Retinal anlage tumor of the epididymis. Most of the tumor is composed of islands of small cells separated by fibrous stroma. Several islands of larger cells full of melanin pigment are also seen.

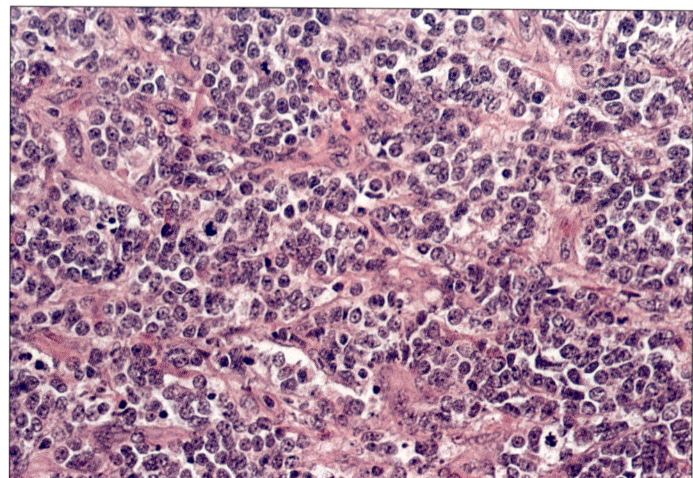

Figure 8.27 Retinal anlage tumor of the epididymis. The small neoplastic cells have scanty cytoplasm and round hyperchromatic nuclei. Two mitotic figures are visible.

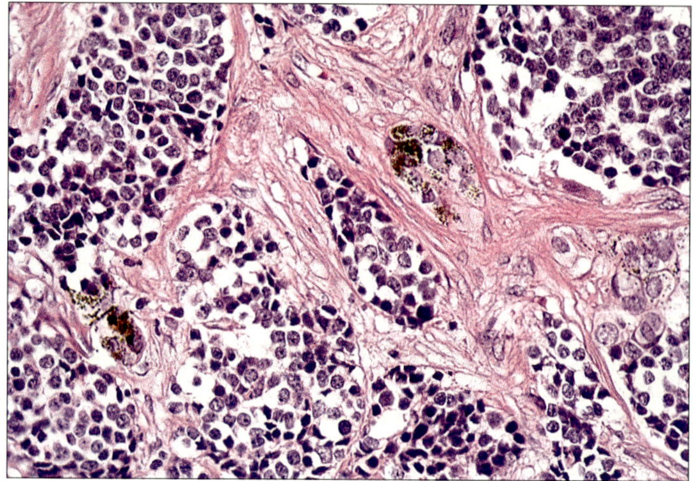

Figure 8.28 Retinal anlage tumor of the epididymis. Some of the large cells are filled with melanin pigment. Other large cells (far right) contain abundant eosinophilic cytoplasm with relatively few pigment granules.

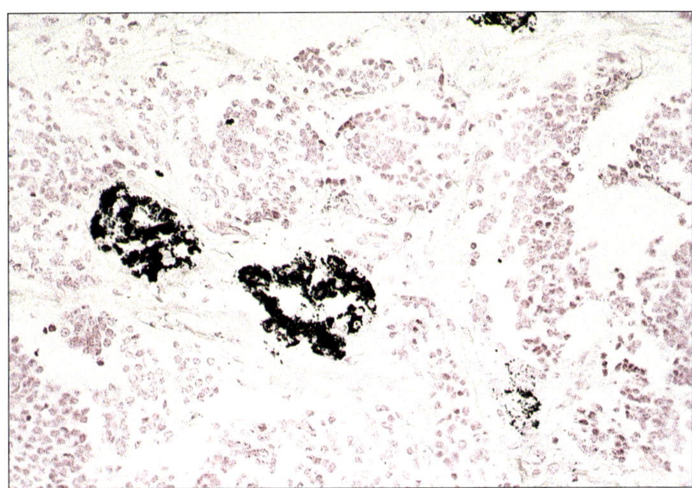

Figure 8.29 Retinal anlage tumor of the epididymis. The large cells are stained for melanin by the Masson-Fontana technique.

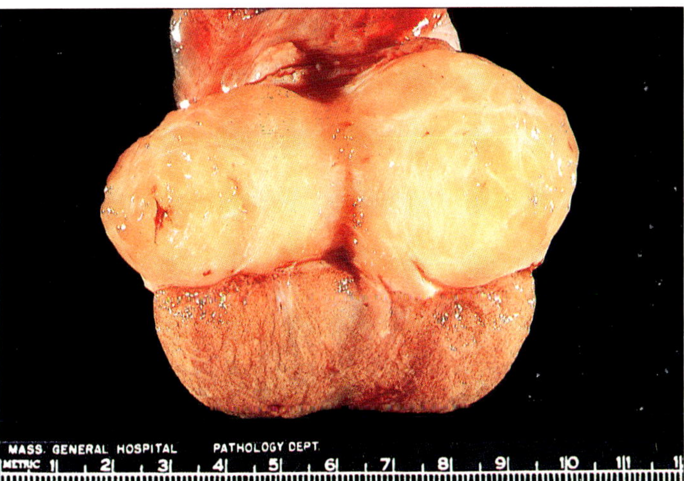

Figure 8.30 Paratesticular neurofibroma. The tumor is pale yellow and streaked with white.

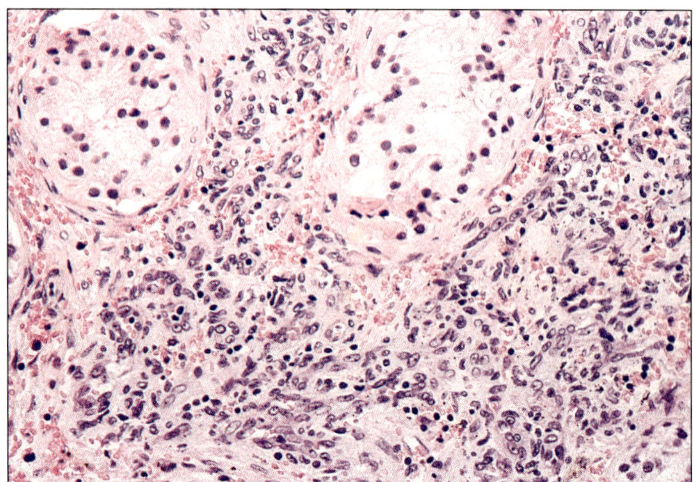

Figure 8.31 Hemangioendothelioma of the testis. The tumor lies in the interstitial tissue and is composed of small capillaries lined by plump endothelial cells.

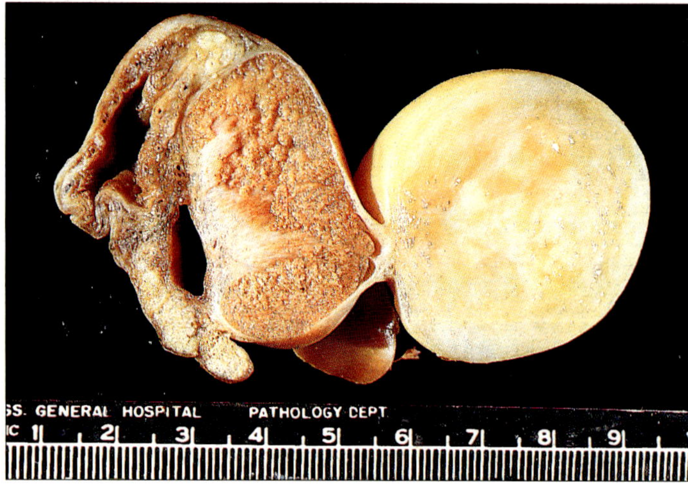

Figure 8.32 Fibroma of the tunica albuginea. The polypoid mass has a flat, pale yellow–white appearance.

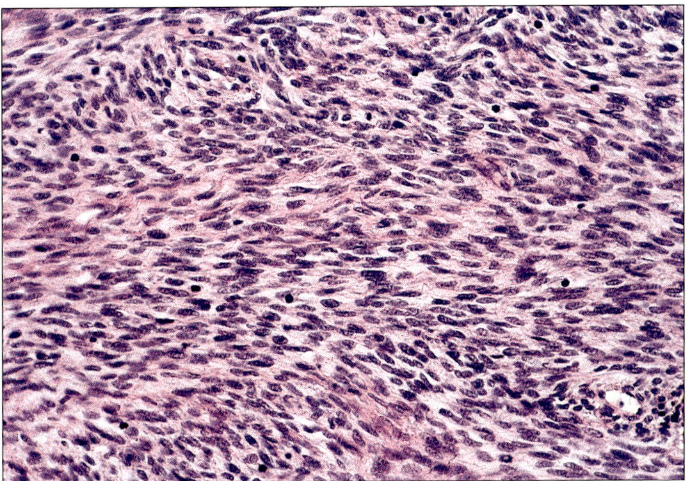

Figure 8.33 Fibrosarcoma of testis. The tumor is composed of closely packed spindle cells. Several mitotic figures are visible.

References

1. Golden A, Ash JE. Adenomatoid tumors of the genital tract. *Am J Pathol* 21:63–79, 1945.
2. Viprakasit D, Tannenbaum M, Smith AM. Adenomatoid tumor of the male genital tract. *Urology* 4:325–327, 1974.
3. Miller F, Lieberman MK. Local invasion in adenomatoid tumors. *Cancer* 21:933–939, 1968.
4. Keily EA, Flanagan A, Williams G. Intrascrotal adenomatoid tumors. *Br J Urol* 60:255–257, 1987.
5. Hartwick RWJ, Srigley JR, Burns B, McCaughey WTE. A clinicopathologic review of 112 paratesticular tumors. *Lab Invest* 56:30A, 1987.
6. Kasdon EJ. Malignant mesothelioma of the tunica vaginalis propria testis: Report of two cases. *Cancer* 23:1144–1150, 1969.
7. Antman K, Cohen S, Dimitrov NV, et al. Malignant mesothelioma of the tunica vaginalis testis. *J Clin Oncol* 2:447–451, 1984.
8. Young RH, Scully RE. Testicular and paratesticular tumors and tumor-like lesions of ovarian common epithelial and müllerian types: A report of four cases and review of the literature. *Am J Clin Pathol* 86:146–152, 1986.
9. Walker AN, Mills SE, Jones PF, Stanley CM. Borderline serous cystadenoma of the tunica vaginalis testis. *Surg Pathol* 1:431–436, 1988.
10. Brito CG, Bloch T, Foster RS, Bihrle R. Testicular papillary cystadenomatous tumor of low malignant potential: A case report and discussion of the literature. *J Urol* 139:378–379, 1988.
11. Axiotis CA. Intratesticular serous papillary cystadenoma of low malignant potential: An ultrastructural and immunohistochemical study suggesting müllerian differentiation. *Am J Surg Pathol* 12:56–63, 1988.
12. Altaffer LF, Dufour DR, Castleberry GM, Steele SM. Coexisting rete testis adenoma and gonadoblastoma. *J Urol* 127:332–335, 1982.
13. Murao T, Tanahashi T. Adenofibroma of the rete testis: A case report with electron microscopy findings. *Acta Pathol Jpn* 38:105–112, 1988.
14. Gisser SD, Nayak S, Kaneko M, Tchertkoff V. Adenocarcinoma of the rete testis: A review of the literature and report of a case with associated asbestosis. *Hum Pathol* 8:219–224, 1977.
15. Nochomovitz LE, Orenstein JM. Adenocarcinoma of the rete testis: Case report, ultrastructural observations, and clinicopathologic correlates. *Am J Surg Pathol* 8:625–634, 1984.
16. Haas GP, Ohorodnik JM, Farah RN. Cystadenocarcinoma of the rete testis. *J Urol* 137:1232–1233, 1987.
17. Nistal M, Paniagua R. Adenomatous hyperplasia of the rete testis. *J Pathol* 154:343–346, 1988.
18. Channer JL, MacIver AG. Glandular changes in the rete testis: Metastatic tumor or adenomatoid hyperplasia? *J Pathol* 157:81–83, 1989.

19. Price EB. Papillary cystadenoma of the epididymis: A clinicopathologic analysis of 20 cases. *Arch Pathol* 91:456–470, 1971.

20. Lamiell JM, Salazar FG, Hsia YE. Von Hippel–Lindau disease affecting 43 members of a single kindred. *Medicine* 68:1–29, 1989.

21. Salm R. Papillary carcinoma of the epididymis. *J Pathol* 97:253–259, 1969.

22. Kuo T-T, Gomez LG. Monstrous epithelial cells in human epididymis and seminal vesicles: A pseudomalignant change. *Am J Surg Pathol* 5:483–490, 1981.

23. Johnson RE, Scheithauer BW, Dahlin DC. Melanotic neuroectodermal tumor of infancy: A review of seven cases. *Cancer* 52:661–666, 1983.

24. Ricketts RR, Majmudarr B. Epididymal melanotic neuroectodermal tumor of infancy. *Hum Pathol* 16:416–420, 1985.

25. Murayama T, Fujita K, Ohashi T, Matsushita T. Melanotic neuroectodermal tumor of the epididymis in infancy: A case report. *J Urol* 141:105–106, 1989.

26. Hargreaves HK, Scully RE, Richie JP. Benign hemangioendothelioma of the testis: Case report with electron microscopic documentation and review of the literature. *Am J Clin Pathol* 77:637–642, 1982.

27. Young RH, Scully RE. Miscellaneous neoplasms and non-neoplastic lesions. In: *Pathology of the Testis and its Adnexa,* Talerman A, Roth LM, eds. *Contemporary Issues in Surgical Pathology,* vol 7. New York, Churchill Livingstone, 1986, chap 5.

28. Loughlin KR, Retik AB, Weinstein HJ, et al. Genitourinary rhabdomyosarcoma in children. *Cancer* 63:1600–1606, 1989.

29. Cecchetto G, Grotto P, De Bernardi B, Indolfi P, et al. Paratesticular rhabdomyosarcoma in childhood: Experience of the Italian Cooperative Study. *Tumori* 74:645–647, 1988.

30. Prince CL. Rhabdomyosarcoma of the testicle. *J Urol* 48:187–195, 1942.

31. Ravich L, Lerman PH, Drabkin JW, Foltin E. Pure testicular rhabdomyosarcoma. *J Urol* 94:596–599, 1965.

32. Yachia P, Auslaender L. Primary leiomyosarcoma of the testis. *J Urol* 141:955–956, 1989.

33. Matthew T. Osteosarcoma of the testis. *Arch Pathol Lab Med* 105:38–39, 1981.

Nonneoplastic Lesions 9

A variety of nonneoplastic lesions may cause enlargement of the testis and have gross or microscopic features simulating those of a testicular or adnexal tumor.

Adrenocortical Rests

Small yellow nodules of ectopic adrenocortical tissue, usually less than 1 cm in diameter, have been found in the spermatic cord, epididymis, rete testis, and tunica albuginea as well as between the epididymis and testis in approximately 10% of infants (Figures 9.1 to 9.3)[1,2]; although they have been encountered occasionally in older individuals, their frequency has not been investigated in that population. Microscopic examination of adrenocortical rests usually reveals encapsulated nodules that typically exhibit the zonation of layers seen in the normal adrenal cortex; occasionally, the rests are unencapsulated (Figure 9.4).

Testicular 'Tumors' of the Adrenogenital Syndrome

Testicular masses composed of steroid-type cells develop in a significant proportion of males with the untreated or inadequately treated adrenogenital syndrome (AGS).[3] These testicular "tumors" of the AGS occur most often in patients with the salt-losing form of the disorder (21-hydroxylase deficiency) that is untreated or inadequately treated.[3] The "tumors" may become evident in childhood or in adult life. Clinical clues to the diagnosis include the presence of the AGS, a family history of it, and bilateral testicular involvement, which is usually synchronous. Laboratory examination reveals the typical findings of the AGS: increased levels of adrenocorticotropic hormone (ACTH), androstenedione, and 17-hydroxyprogesterone in the plasma and elevated levels of 17-ketosteroids and pregnanetriol in the urine. Other characteristic features are enlargement of the testicular masses and increased hormonal secretion after the administration of ACTH, and a decrease in their size and hormone output after suppression of the elevated ACTH level by the administration of corticosteroids. A few patients with Nelson's syndrome (development of an ACTH-secreting pituitary tumor, typically accompanied by cutaneous hyperpigmentation, after bilateral adrenalectomy for Cushing's disease) have had testicular "tumors," paratesticular "tumors," or both that have resembled those associated with the AGS.[3]

The testicular "tumors" of the AGS, which range up to 10 cm in diameter, appear to originate in the hilar region and extend peripherally into the parenchyma. Sectioning typically reveals dark brown, lobulated tissue traversed by fibrous septa (Figure 9.5). Microscopic examination discloses a diffuse proliferation of large cells resembling Leydig cells (Figure 9.6). These cells have abundant eosinophilic cytoplasm, which typically contains a large amount of lipochrome pigment, but lacks crystals of Reinke (Figure 9.7). Some lesions may exhibit hyaline fibrosis of the stroma (Figure 9.6). Rarely, the nuclei are atypical and abnormal mitotic figures are encountered exceptionally (Figure 9.8). The nature of the lesional cells remains in doubt. Some investigators contend that they are derived from adrenocortical rests, others, that they are Leydig cells that have been "captured" by ACTH, and still others, that they originate from testicular stromal cells that are capable of differentiating into either Leydig or adrenocortical cells depending on the nature of the tropic stimulation.

Although they closely resemble Leydig cell tumors pathologically, testicular "tumors" of the AGS differ from the former in several respects. First, their usual bilaterality contrasts with the exceptional bilaterality of Leydig cell tumors. Second, they are typically dark brown, whereas Leydig cell tumors are more often yellow or yellow-tan. Seminiferous tubules may be present within a testicular "tumor" of the AGS but are found only rarely within a Leydig cell tumor. The cells of the former tend to be larger and to have more abundant cytoplasm than those of the latter and contain lipochrome pigment more frequently and in greater amounts; the presence of this pigment is responsible for the dark color of the lesion on gross examination; crystals of Reinke have not been identified within the cells of the testicular "tumors" of the AGS, but are found in 35% to 40% of diagnosable Leydig cell tumors.

Cysts

Epidermoid cysts account for approximately 1% of testicular enlargements. They occur at all ages, but are most common during the second to fourth decades.[4,5] They average 2 cm in diameter, are round to oval, and are composed of laminated cheesy material surrounded by a fibrous wall (Figure 9.9). Microscopic examination shows that at least part of the cyst wall is lined by keratinizing squamous epithelium (Figure 9.10); the lining may be denuded over large areas, with ulceration and foreign body giant cell reaction. It is important to sample epidermoid cysts extensively to exclude teratomatous elements, an association with intratubular or invasive germ cell neoplasia, or an adjacent scar; any of these findings, if present, warrants the diagnosis of teratoma.

Other types of testicular cyst are extremely rare; they include parenchymal cysts of undetermined origin lined by cuboidal or flattened epithelium, and cysts arising from the mesothelium of the tunica albuginea. True hermaphrodites who are phenotypic males may have ovotestes or, very rarely, an ovary in the scrotum.[6] The ovarian tissue may contain cystic follicles and corpora lutea, and on occasion, ovulation causes the sudden onset of hemorrhage with pain and a mass in the scrotum simulating a testicular tumor.

Cystic Dysplasia

This rare lesion, which occurs in infants and children, is characterized by the presence of multiple anastomosing cysts of varying sizes and shapes, separated by fibrous septa.[7–9] There have been three reported cases associated with ipsilateral renal agenesis and one with bilateral renal dysplasia.[7,8] The lesion was bilateral in two of the seven reported cases. Gross examination reveals a multicystic mass replacing most of the testis (Figure 9.11). The process begins in the region of the rete and extends into the parenchyma, which may be compressed to form a thin rim. The cysts are lined by a single layer of flat or cuboidal epithelial cells (Figure 9.12), which have been shown by ultrastructural studies to be similar to those of the rete testis.[9]

Nodular Precocious Maturation

Rarely, gonadotropin-induced or gonadotropin-independent sexual precocity, instead of being characterized by diffuse bilateral testicular enlargement, is associated with unilateral nodular enlargement simulating a neoplasm. In such cases, there are variable degrees of maturation of tubules and Leydig cells within the ill-defined nodule and little or no maturation in the adjacent testis (Figures 9.13, 9.14). We have seen one such case in association with an extragonadal hCG-producing germ cell tumor.

Orchitis

Bacterial

An orchidectomy is occasionally performed in cases in which the testis is involved by bacterial infection. The epididymis is typically also affected in such cases and the gross appearance varies, depending on the relative extents of epididymal and testicular involvement and the chronicity of the process. The testis may contain abscesses or be fibrotic and adherent to adjacent tissues. Rarely, a neoplasm is suggested in long-standing cases.[10] Microscopic examination discloses varying amounts of acute and chronic inflammation, abscess formation, granulation tissue, and fibrosis, depending on the duration of the process. In some cases there is focal infarction, which may be the result of venous occlusion.[11]

Viral

The best-known form of viral orchitis is caused by the mumps virus,[12] but a wide variety of other viruses have also been implicated, most often the Coxsackie B virus.[13] The testis is involved in approximately one fourth of adult males with mumps, but in well under 1% of children with this disease. Testicular involvement is bilateral in almost one fifth of the cases and is accompanied by epididymitis in 85% of the cases.[14] On clinical examination the testis is swollen and tender. Incision of the tunica albuginea reveals edema and, in some cases, hemorrhage. Microscopic examination discloses interstitial edema early in the course, followed by vascular dilatation and interstitial lymphocytic infiltration.[12] Subsequently, interstitial hemorrhage occurs, accompanied by inflammatory cell infiltration of the seminiferous tubules and degeneration of the germinal epithelium

(Figure 9.15). Healing results in patchy hyalinization of tubules and interstitial fibrosis, with intervening areas of normal testis. The microscopic features of other rarely described forms of viral orchitis resemble those of mumps orchitis (Figures 9.16, 9.17). In the exceptional cases in which mumps orchitis precedes parotitis or is the sole evidence of the infection, or in those cases in which orchitis is the exclusive or major manifestation of another viral illness, the gross and microscopic findings may be confused with those of a malignant tumor, particularly a seminoma or lymphoma. Careful examination of the cellular infiltrate, however, enables one to make the correct diagnosis.

Granulomatous

Infectious. Tuberculosis, leprosy, syphilis, and various fungal infections may cause granulomatous inflammation of the testis. In tuberculosis the epididymis is the primary site of the disease (Figure 9.18) and the testis is usually affected only in the late stages (Figure 9.19).[15,16] This sequence of involvement, the 30% frequency of bilaterality, and the 50% frequency of an abscess or sinus tract are important clues to the infectious nature of the process.

Testicular involvement is very common in patients with lepromatous leprosy. Leprosy, in contrast to tuberculosis, involves the testis more commonly than the epididymis. Both testes are usually affected; they are typically normal or decreased in size, but are occasionally enlarged. The microscopic findings have been divided into three stages: vascular, characterized by thickening of vessel walls and a perivascular inflammatory infiltrate; interstitial, with progressive obliterative endarteritis and interstitial fibrosis; and obliterative, with loss of the normal architecture of the testis and replacement of its parenchyma by fibrous tissue.[17] Lepra bacilli can usually be identified during the first two stages.

The testis may be involved in congenital syphilis and in the late secondary and tertiary stages of acquired syphilis.[18] In congenital syphilis, bilateral painless testicular enlargement is usually present, and microscopic examination shows interstitial inflammation, which may be granulomatous, endarteritis, and fibrosis. A similar appearance also characterizes involvement by tertiary syphilis, but in the latter disorder, gummas of varying sizes may also be encountered (Figures 9.20, 9.21). On very rare occasions fungal and parasitic diseases involve the testis.[14]

Idiopathic. Idiopathic granulomatous orchitis[19,20] is one of the commoner forms of nonneoplastic testicular enlargement, accounting for 0.2%

of testicular masses.[14] The lesion, which usually occurs during the fifth or sixth decade,[19] follows a urinary tract infection with gram-negative bacilli in approximately two thirds of the cases. The testis enlarges sometimes with pain or tenderness, which may disappear, leaving a painless mass.[19] The contralateral testis is metachronously affected in occasional cases. Although granulomatous orchitis may be clinically indistinguishable from a neoplasm in some cases, in other cases, the history of symptoms consistent with a flu-like illness, the sudden onset of testicular swelling, and the associated pain or tenderness suggest an inflammatory process.

Gross examination reveals replacement of the testicular parenchyma by homogeneous, sometimes lobulated, tan-yellow, gray or white tissue (Figure 9.22). The process is usually diffuse but a localized, well-circumscribed nodule is sometimes encountered. The epididymis and spermatic cord are involved in approximately one half of the cases and an exudate is often present on the tunica vaginalis. Microscopic examination shows filling of the seminiferous tubules by inflammatory cells, among which epithelioid histiocytes predominate (Figure 9.23); Langhans'-type giant cells are seen in one third of the cases (Figure 9.24). The interstitial tissue contains numerous chronic inflammatory cells, including eosinophils in most of the cases. The primarily intratubular location of the granulomatous process is helpful in differentiating the lesion from granulomatous orchitis of infectious origin and from the very rare sarcoidosis of the testis, in both of which the granulomas are predominantly interstitial. Also, necrosis within the granulomas may be seen in the infectious lesions, but not in idiopathic granulomatous orchitis. Identification of organisms by smear or culture is the most effective way to confirm or exclude specific forms of granulomatous orchitis. It should be emphasized, however, that remnants of sperm may also be acid-fast in cases of idiopathic granulomatous orchitis.[14]

Sarcoidosis may affect the epididymis and, rarely, the testis[21]; exceptionally, testicular enlargement caused by this disorder has resulted in an orchidectomy.[14]

Malakoplakia

There are almost 40 reported cases in which malakoplakia, an inflammatory disorder that is most common in the urinary tract but that may occur in any organ or tissue, has involved the testis, epididymis, or both.[22] The testis alone is affected in approximately two thirds of the cases, and the epididymis alone is affected on rare occasions. The symptoms are nonspecific; occasionally, there is a history of a urinary tract infection. The involved testis is usually enlarged and may be difficult to remove because of fibrous adhesions to surrounding tissues. In all of the reported cases, testicular enlargement has been unilateral and has occurred in an adult.

Sectioning shows replacement of all or part of the testicular parenchyma by yellow, tan, or brown tissue, which is often divided into lobules by bands of fibrous tissue (Figure 9.25); the tissue is usually soft, but may be firm if there is a significant amount of fibrosis. The frequent finding of one or more abscesses is a strong clue to the diagnosis (Figure 9.25), as is the presence of reactive inflammatory changes in the tunica albuginea and involvement of the epididymis, which may become firm and fibrotic. Microscopic examination reveals replacement of the tubules and interstitial tissue by large histiocytes with abundant granular eosinophilic cytoplasm (von Hansemann cells) (Figures 9.26 to 9.28), some of which contain solid and targetoid basophilic inclusions of varying sizes (Michaelis-Gutmann bodies) (Figure 9.29).[23] Acute and chronic inflammatory cells, granulation tissue, and fibrosis are also present and may obscure the characteristic features of the process, especially if Michaelis-Gutmann bodies are inconspicuous. These structures are accentuated by PAS (Figure 9.30), von Kossa (Figure 9.31), and iron stains (Figure 9.32), for which almost all cases are positive. Ultrastructural studies have shown that the Michaelis-Gutmann bodies are phagolysosomes that have ingested the breakdown products of bacteria of various types, most often *Escherichia coli*.[22] As discussed earlier (see page 103), malakoplakia is sometimes confused with a Leydig cell tumor, but the latter does not involve tubules and its cells lack the characteristic features of von Hansemann cells.

Fibromatous Periorchitis (Fibrous Pseudotumor) (Nodular Periorchitis)

In the diffuse form of this disorder, dense fibrous tissue involves the tunica vaginalis, and in the localized form, single or disseminated plaques or nodules may be present (Figure 9.33).[14,24] Sectioning reveals firm white tissue and microscopic examination typically demonstrates hyalinized collagen, which may be focally calcified (Figure 9.34); in some cases the lesion is more cellular, with inflammation and granulation tissue. This disorder is generally believed to be reactive.

Cholesterol Granuloma and Calcification of Tunica Vaginalis

Rarely, a foreign body reaction to cholesterol crystals in the tunica vaginalis produces a firm mass that may suggest a testicular or paratesticular tumor.[25] Diffuse calcification of the tunica vaginalis visible on x-ray examination has also been reported.[14]

Sclerosing Lipogranuloma

A granulomatous mass resulting from the injection of lipids to enhance the size of the genitalia is rarely encountered. The mass is usually peripheral to the testis, but occasionally involves it as well.[26] The presence of a hard mass may lead to orchidectomy. Gross examination reveals an ill-defined, firm, oily mass, and microscopic examination discloses lipid vacuoles of varying size surrounded by foreign-body giant cells, with chronic inflammation and fibrosis that is often extensive and may be hyaline (Figures 9.35, 9.36).

Splenic-Gonadal Fusion

In this unusual abnormality, which has a strong male predilection, splenic and gonadal tissues become adherent and fuse during early intrauterine development.[27–29] The left testis is almost invariably involved. The abnormality occurs in two forms, continuous and discontinuous.[27] In the continuous form a cord connects the splenic tissue to the testis, while in the discontinuous form no cord is present. Small aggregates of splenic tissue may be found in the cord as it traverses the peritoneal cavity, or the cord may be composed entirely of splenic tissue. Almost one third of the patients with the continuous form have severe defects of the extremities (peromelia), sometimes associated with micrognathia.[27] In patients without associated congenital abnormalities the clinical presentation is in the form of a scrotal or inguinal mass. The latter may be discovered during an operation for an inguinal hernia, which is present in more than one third of the cases, or during an operation on an undescended testis, which is present in approximately one sixth of the cases. Two patients were reported to have had pain in the scrotum associated with attacks of malaria.[14]

The splenic tissue attached to the testis typically forms a discrete mass, which is usually small, but may be as large as 12 cm. It is almost always fused to the upper pole of the testis or the head of the epididymis, but occasionally it is attached to the lower pole and rarely it is intratesticular (Figure 9.37). The gross and microscopic features of the lesion are similar to those of a normal spleen (Figure 9.38).

Infarcts and Hematomas

A testicular infarct (Figure 9.39) may be caused by thrombotic vascular occlusion or torsion.[30] Occasionally, a testicular infarct simulates a neoplasm on clinical examination (Figure 9.40). The sectioned surfaces of an infarct may be hemorrhagic or pale (Figure 9.39). Microscopic examination typically shows necrotic tubules and varying degrees of hemorrhage (Figure 9.41). Although testicular hemorrhage is usually related to a malignant neoplasm, rupture of an artery involved by arteritis rarely leads to the formation of a large hematoma, which may be confused on gross examination with a choriocarcinoma (Figure 9.42). Testicular vasculitis may be accompanied by, or followed by, evidence of systemic vasculitis, but it may also occur as an isolated phenomenon (Figure 9.41).[31] In cases of periarteritis nodosa, in which testicular involvement is common, infarcts may also be seen.[32]

Sperm Granuloma of the Epididymis and Vas Deferens

In this lesion, which almost always involves the epididymis or vas deferens,[33,34] a granulomatous reaction to extravasated sperm produces a painful nodule, which may measure up to 4 cm in its greatest dimension and has occasionally been mistaken for a testicular tumor. Sperm granulomas are now related to a prior vasectomy in over 40% of the cases.[14] Approximately 90% of sperm granulomas that follow vasectomy are in the vas deferens and the remainder are in the epididymis.[12] On gross examination sperm granulomas are typically firm but may have small, soft yellow to white foci on sectioning. The microscopic appearance varies, depending on the stage of the process. In the initial phase there is an infiltrate of neutrophils, which is gradually replaced by epithelioid histiocytes; the histiocytes surround the sperm and their presence results in the most characteristic appearance of the lesion (Figures 9.43, 9.44); calcification is occasionally seen. In the later stages of the lesion there is progressive fibrosis and hyalinization, and lipochrome pigment deposition may be prominent. Sperm granulomas occurring in the vas are associated with vasitis nodosa in approximately one third of the cases (Figure 9.45). Microscopic examination reveals small glandlike structures lined by cuboidal epithelium in the wall of the vas and in the surrounding connective tissue.[35–37] Neural invasion may be observed.[37] This distinctive lesion should not be confused with primary or metastatic adenocarcinoma.

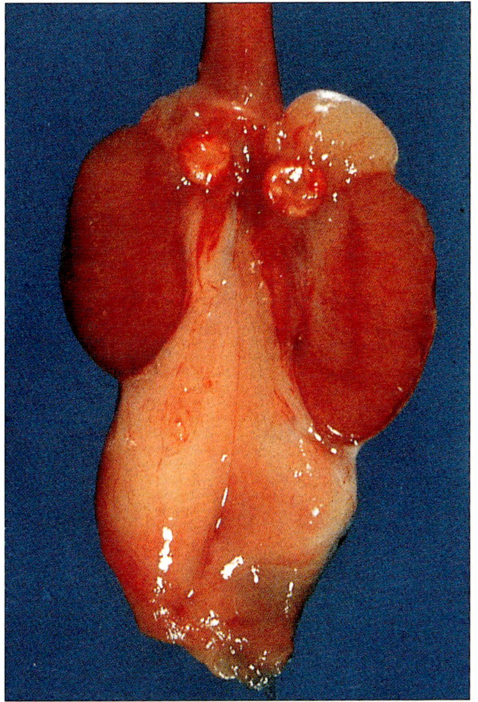

Figure 9.1 Adrenocortical rest, paratesticular. A small, round, orange-yellow nodule lies between the testis and epididymis. (Courtesy of Dr Ernest Lack.)

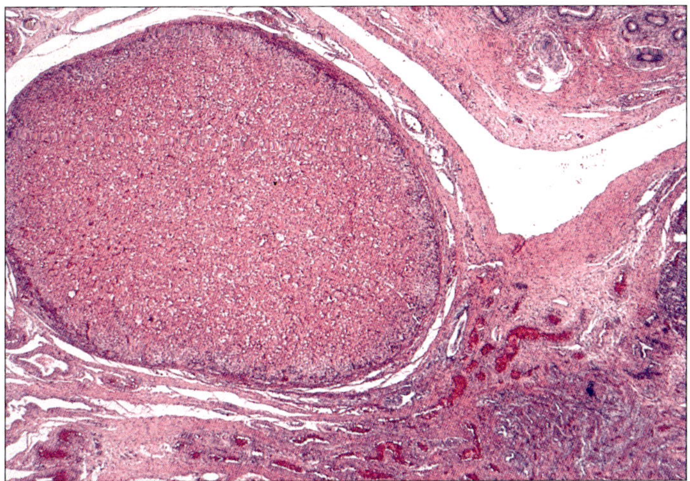

Figure 9.2 Adrenocortical rest. The large encapsulated nodule is composed principally of fetal cortex. (Courtesy of Dr Ernest Lack.)

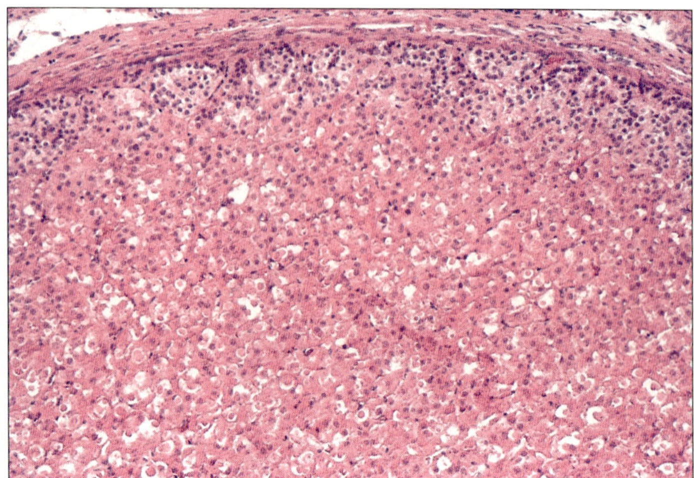

Figure 9.3 Adrenocortical rest. Most of the cells are of the fetal cortical type. A thin layer of definitive cortex is present just beneath the capsule. (Courtesy of Dr Ernest Lack.)

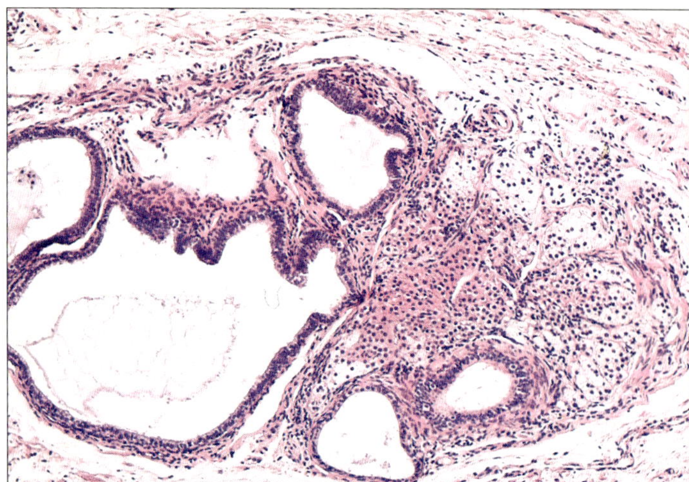

Figure 9.4 Adrenocortical rest in the epididymis. This structure is unencapsulated and is composed of centrally located cells containing abundant eosinophilic cytoplasm as well as vacuolated cells resembling those of the zona glomerulosa at the periphery.

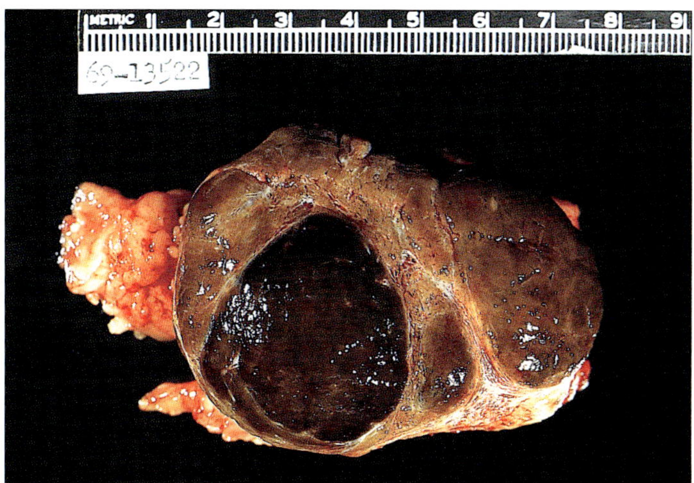

Figure 9.5 Testicular "tumor" of the adrenogenital syndrome. The mass is composed of multiple brown to almost black nodules separated by fibrous septa.

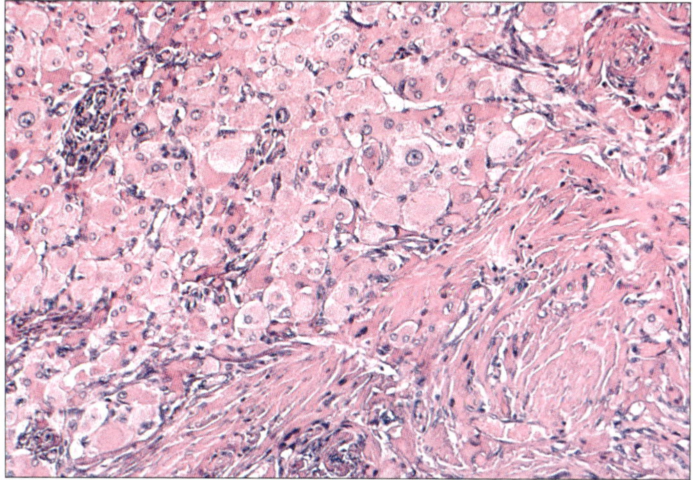

Figure 9.6 Testicular "tumor" of the adrenogenital syndrome. The cells are large and contain abundant eosinophilic cytoplasm and central nuclei, some of which have prominent nucleoli. Extensive hyaline fibrosis is present.

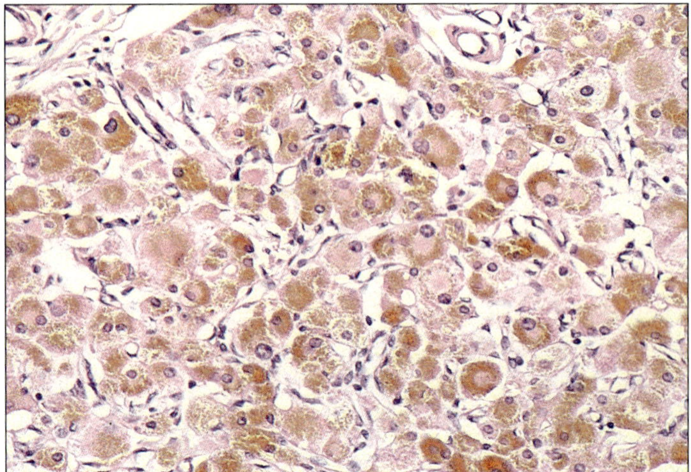

Figure 9.7 Testicular "tumor" of the adrenogenital syndrome. The cells contain large quantities of brown-yellow lipochrome pigment in their cytoplasm.

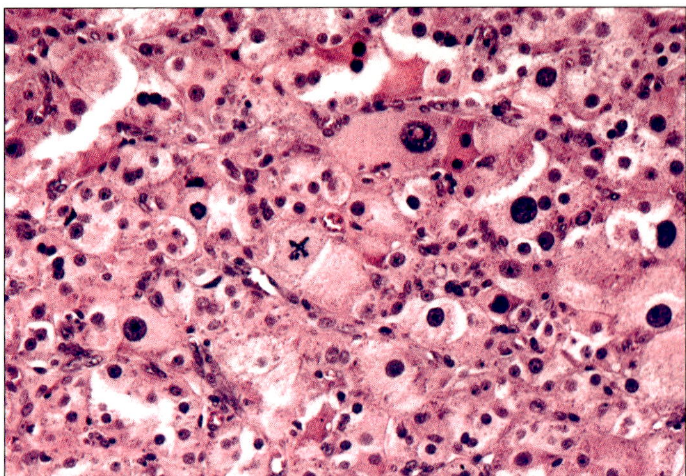

Figure 9.8 Testicular "tumor" of the adrenogenital syndrome. Many of the nuclei are large and hyperchromatic. A tetrapolar mitotic figure is present.

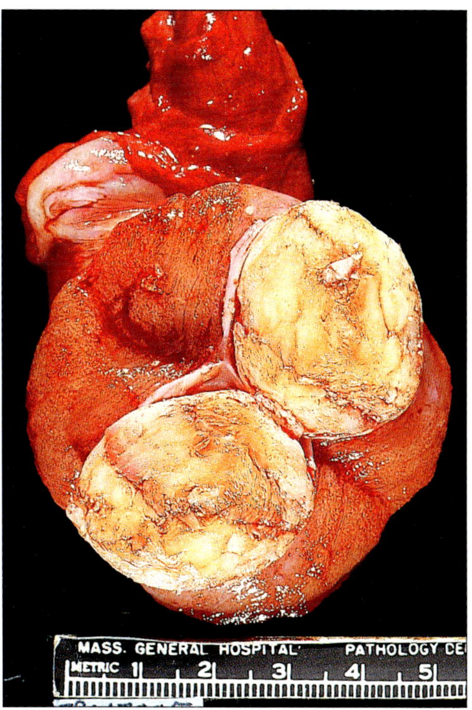

Figure 9.9 Epidermoid cyst. A thin-walled cyst is filled with cheesy, keratinous material.

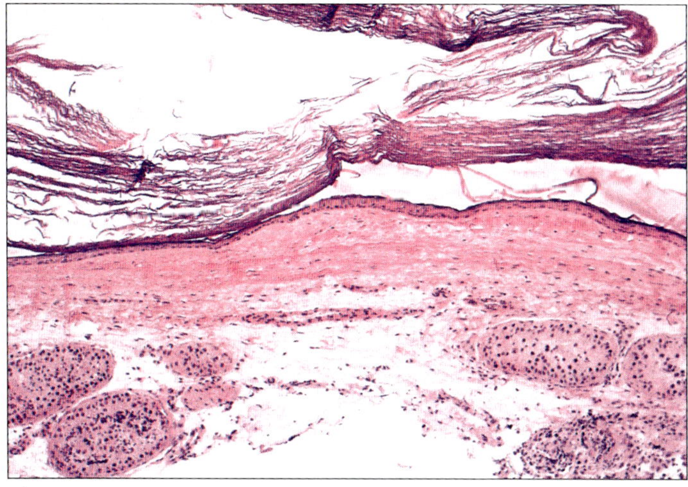

Figure 9.10 Epidermoid cyst. The cyst is lined by keratinizing squamous epithelium with keratin in the lumen.

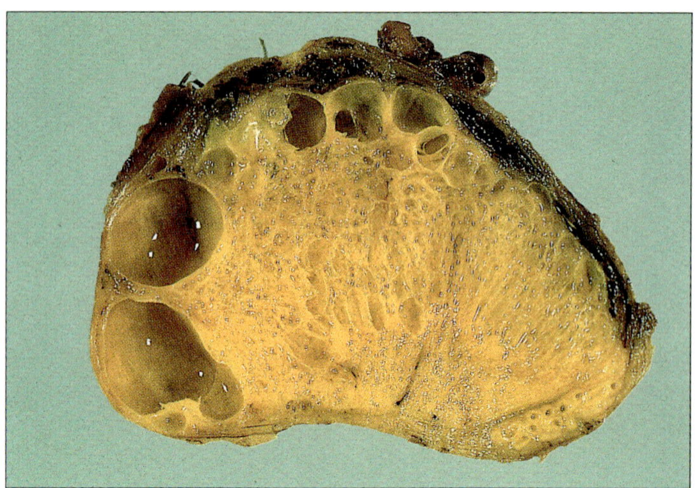

Figure 9.11 Cystic dysplasia. Multiple cysts of varying sizes are visible. (Courtesy of Professor W. Wegmann.)

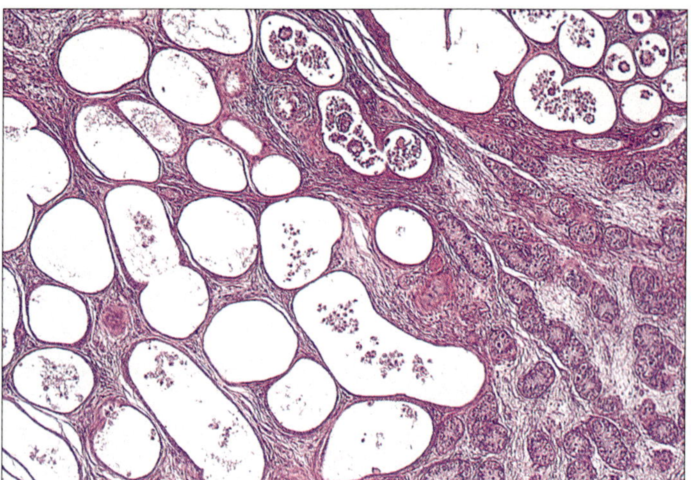

Figure 9.12 Cystic dysplasia. Most of the tubules are cystically dilated and lined by flattened epithelium. (Courtesy of Professor W. Wegmann.)

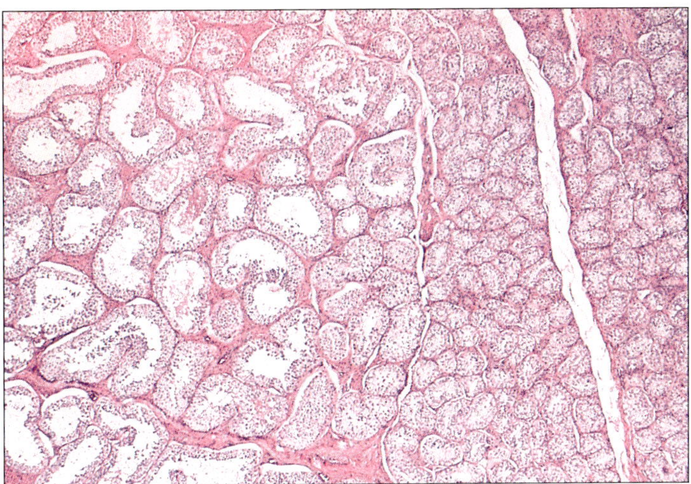

Figure 9.13 Nodular precocious maturation. The nodule is composed of mature testicular tissue, and the uninvolved testis on the left side has the appearance of normal prepubertal testis. This boy had an extratesticular, hCG-secreting, germ cell tumor.

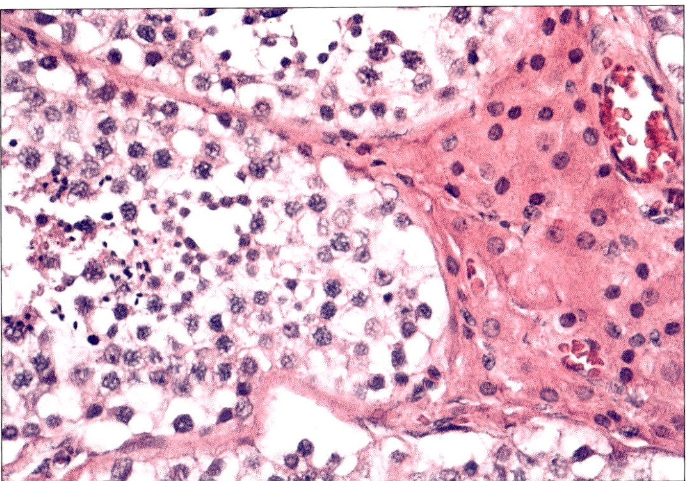

Figure 9.14 Nodular precocious maturation. The tissue in the nodule is composed of mature tubules containing spermatozoa, and hyperplastic Leydig cells.

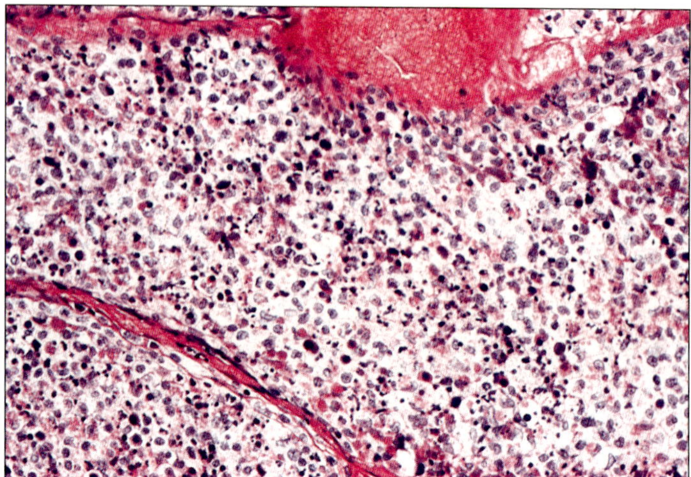

Figure 9.15 Mumps orchitis. The tubules are distended by mononuclear cells, polymorphonuclear leukocytes, degenerating cells, and nuclear debris.

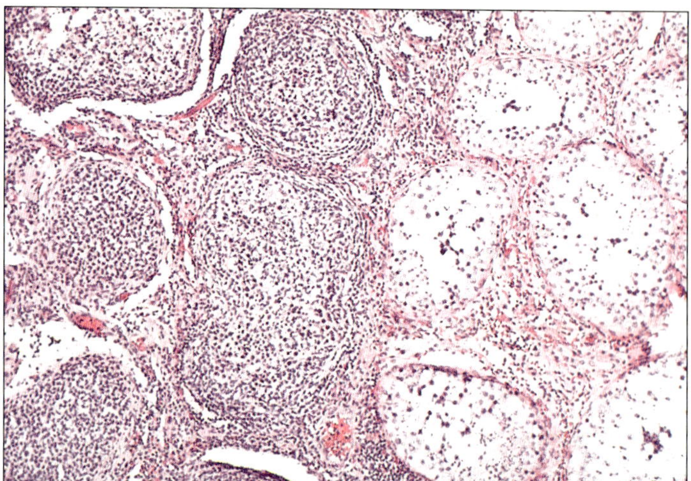

Figure 9.16 Orchitis, probably viral. Many of the tubules are distended by mononuclear cells. There is also extensive mononuclear cell infiltration of the interstitial tissue.

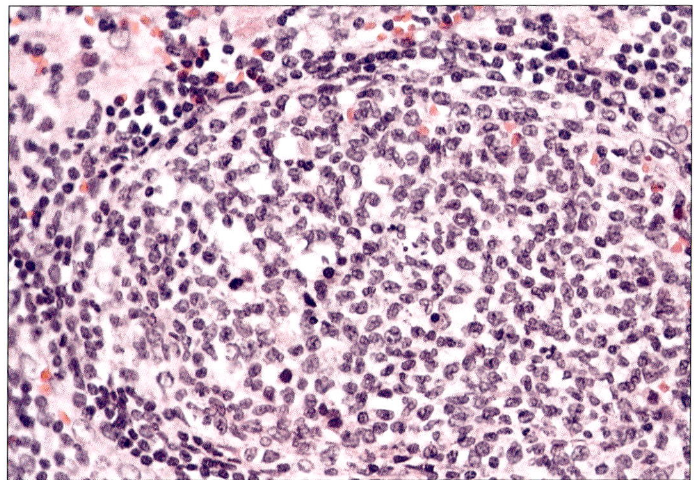

Figure 9.17 Orchitis, probably viral. A tubule is distended by mononuclear cells and surrounded by lymphocytes.

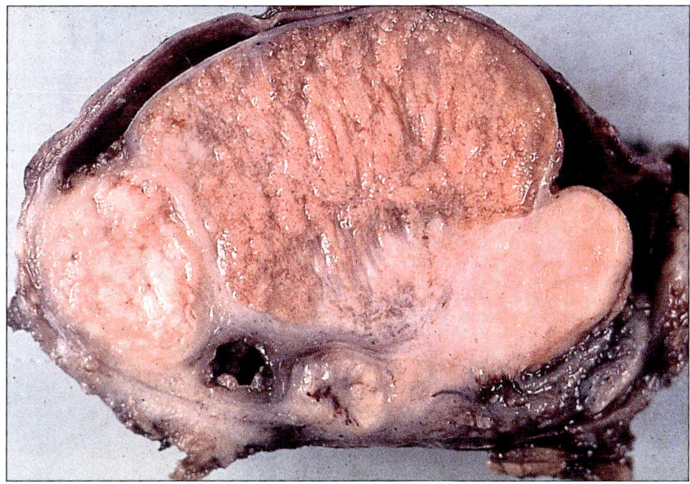

Figure 9.18 Tuberculous epididymo-orchitis. There is extensive nodular involvement of the entire epididymis with secondary involvement of the testis. (Courtesy of Professor D. O'B. Hourihane.)

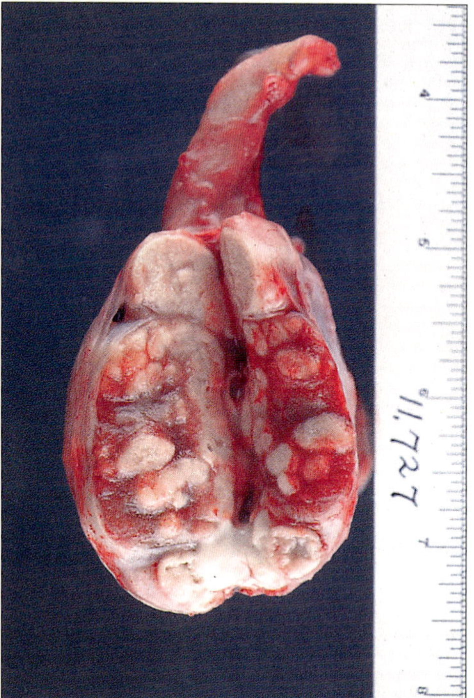

Figure 9.19 Tuberculous epididymoorchitis. Multiple caseous nodules are present in the epididymis and testis.

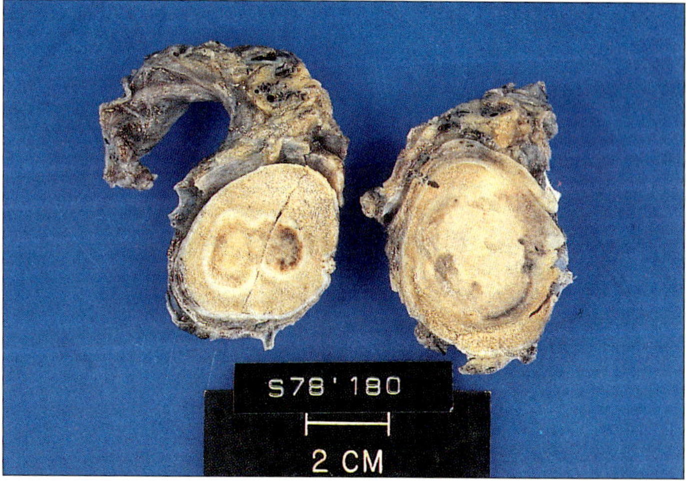

Figure 9.20 Syphilitic gumma of testis. A large area of necrotic tissue is surrounded by a rim of white tissue.

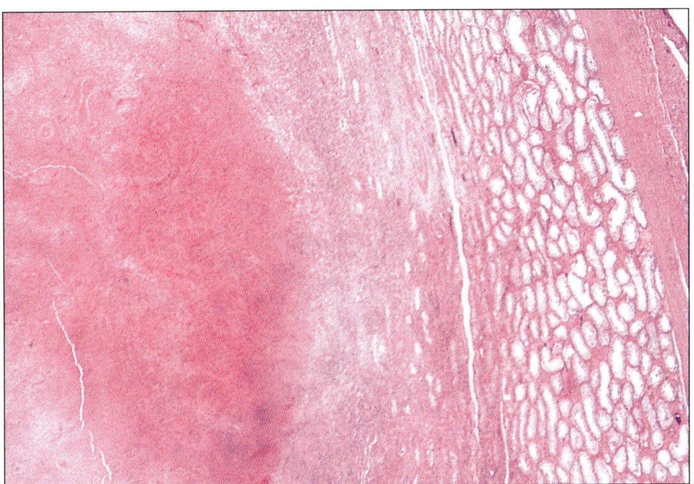

Figure 9.21 Syphilitic gumma of testis. An area of gummatous necrosis is bordered by a zone of fibrous tissue containing many chronic inflammatory cells.

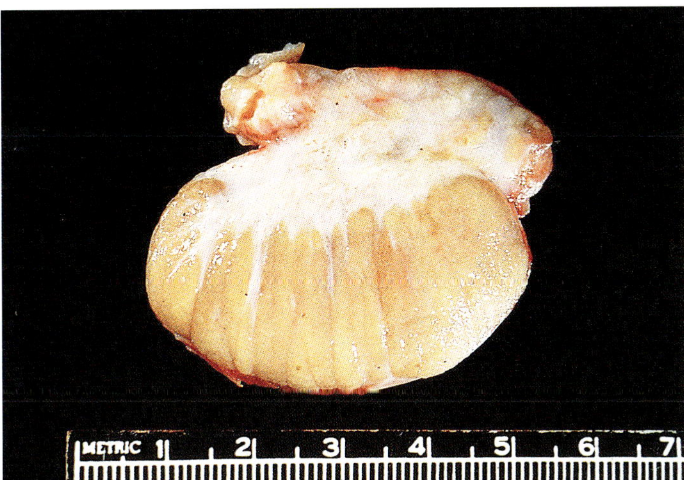

Figure 9.22 Granulomatous orchitis, idiopathic. The parenchyma is replaced by lobulated, pale-yellow tissue.

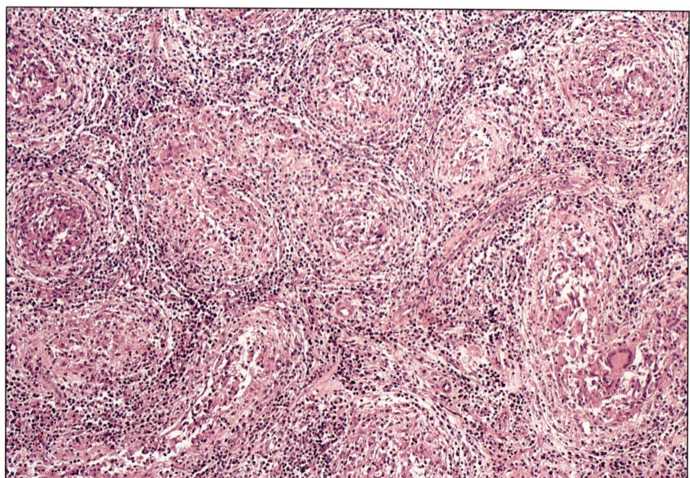

Figure 9.23 Granulomatous orchitis, idiopathic. The tubules have been largely replaced by epithelioid cells and round cells. There is extensive round cell infiltration of the interstitial tissue. A Langhans'-type giant cell is seen at the right.

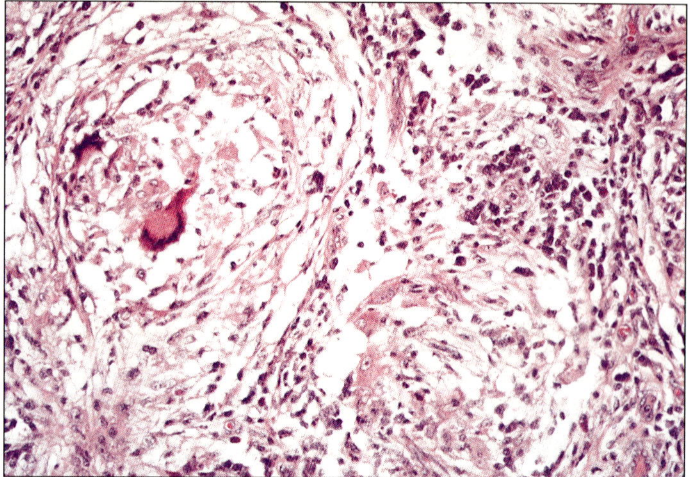

Figure 9.24 Granulomatous orchitis. Several tubules contain epithelioid cells. Two Langhans' giant cells are visible.

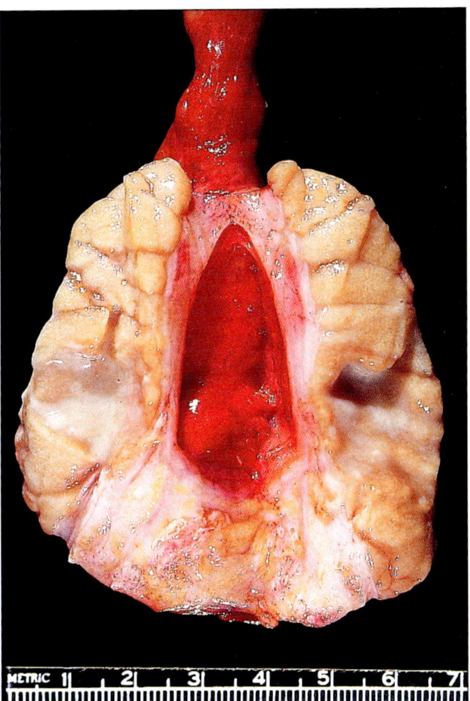

Figure 9.25 Malakoplakia of the testis. The parenchyma has been replaced by lobulated, pale yellow tissue. An abscess containing cream-colored purulent exudate is present.

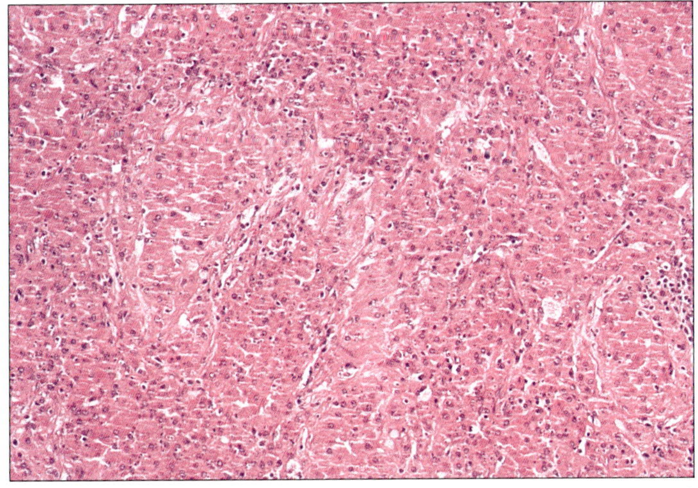

Figure 9.26 Malakoplakia of the testis. Both tubules and interstitial tissue are replaced by large epithelioid cells with abundant eosinophilic cytoplasm (von Hansemann cells).

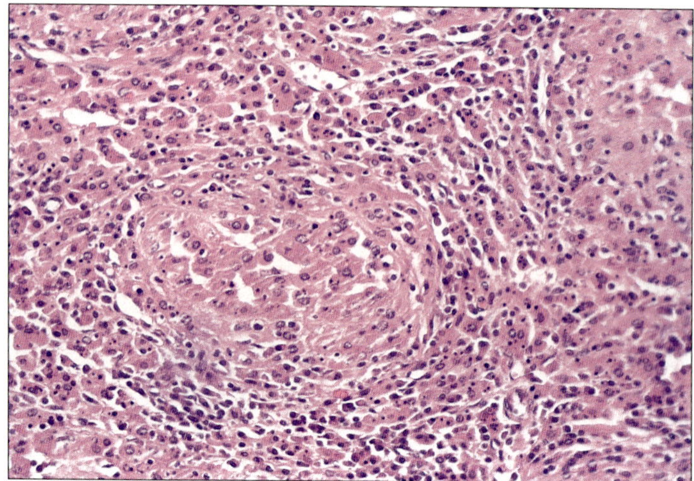

Figure 9.27 Malakoplakia of the testis. The tubules are filled with von Hansemann cells and round cells. The interstitial tissue contains similar cells, including numerous round cells.

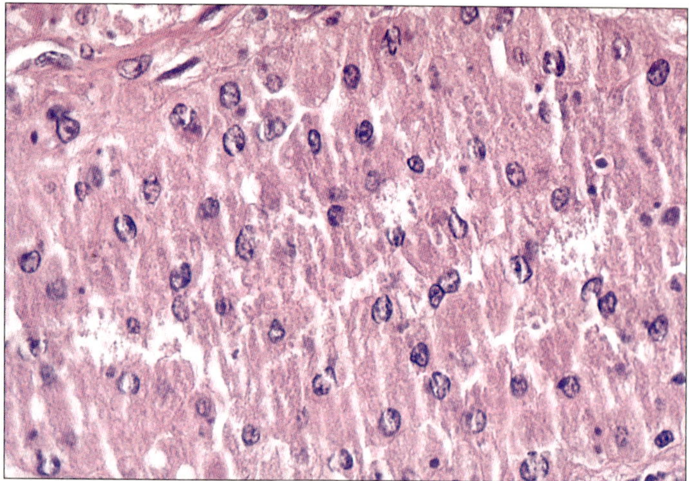

Figure 9.28 Malakoplakia of the testis. Intratubular von Hansemann cells contain abundant, coarsely granular cytoplasm.

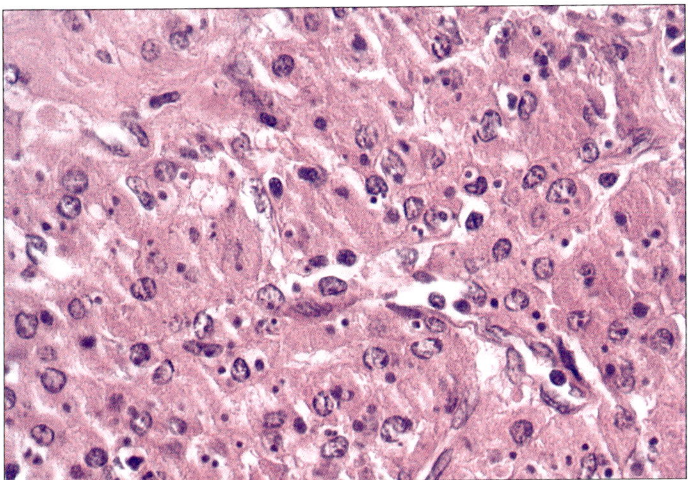

Figure 9.29 Malakoplakia of the testis. The von Hansemann cells contain numerous Michaelis-Gutmann bodies, characterized by basophilic staining and variation in size, and sometimes by clear halos.

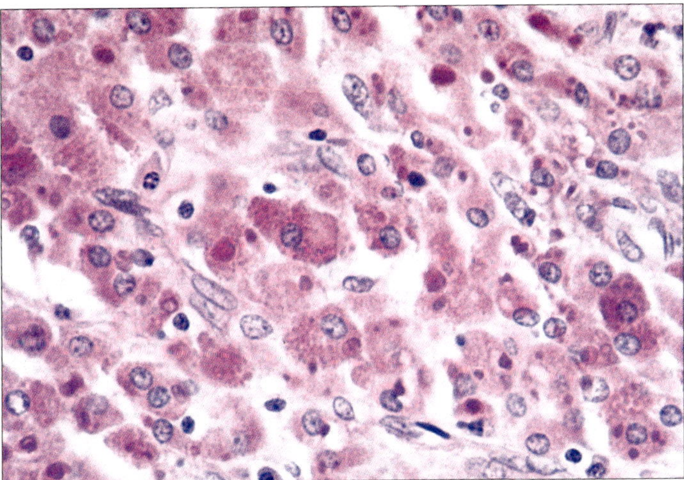

Figure 9.30 Malakoplakia of the testis. The granules of the von Hansemann cells and the Michaelis-Gutmann bodies are stained by the PAS technique.

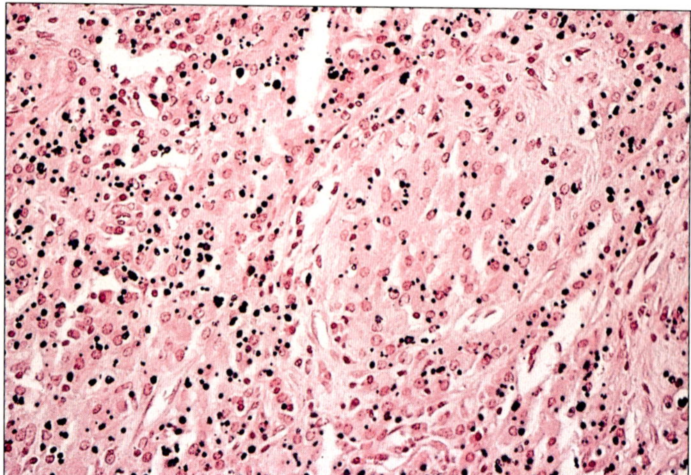

Figure 9.31 Malakoplakia of the testis. The Michaelis-Gutmann bodies are stained for (calcium) phosphate by the von Kossa technique.

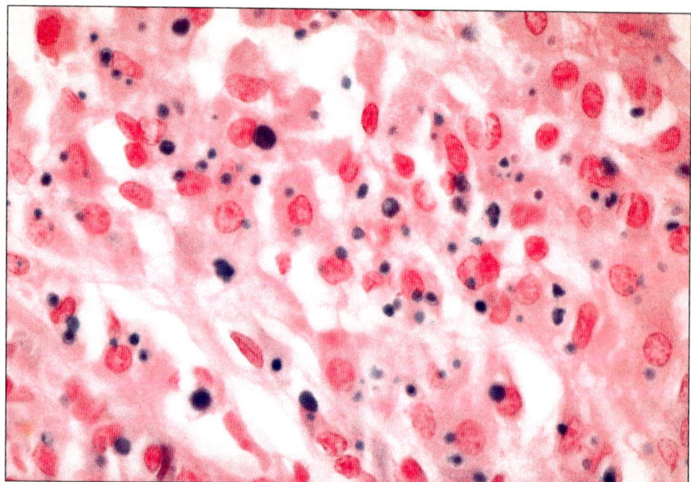

Figure 9.32 Malakoplakia of the testis. The Michaelis-Gutmann bodies are stained for iron by the Prussian blue technique.

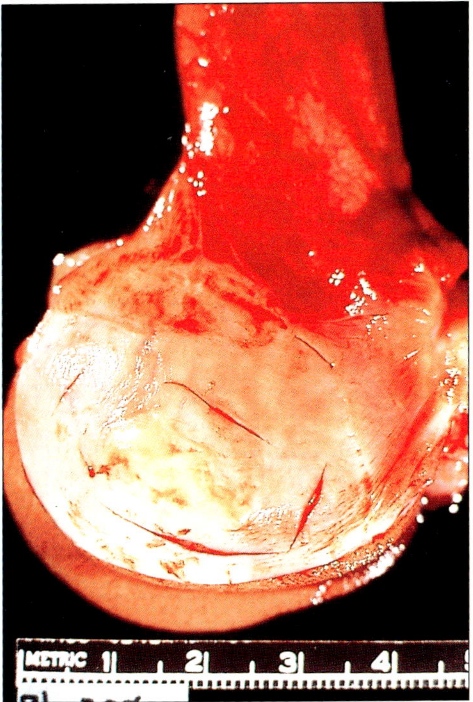

Figure 9.33 Fibromatous periorchitis. A localized, pale yellow thickening of the tunica albuginea is surrounded by four incisions.

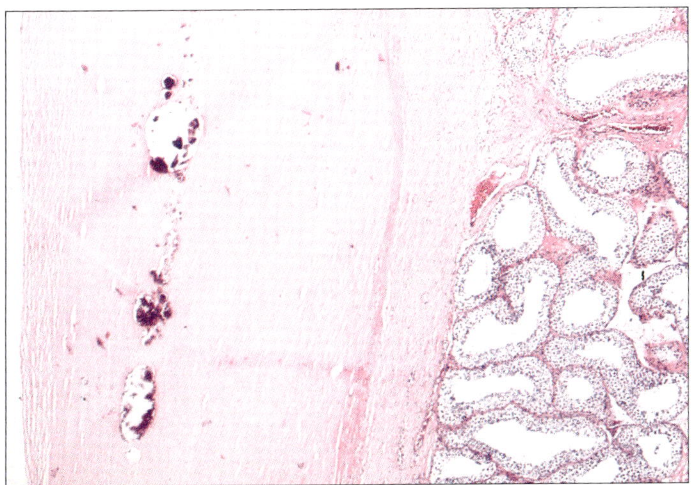

Figure 9.34 Fibromatous periorchitis. The tunica albuginea is thick, hyalinized, and focally calcified.

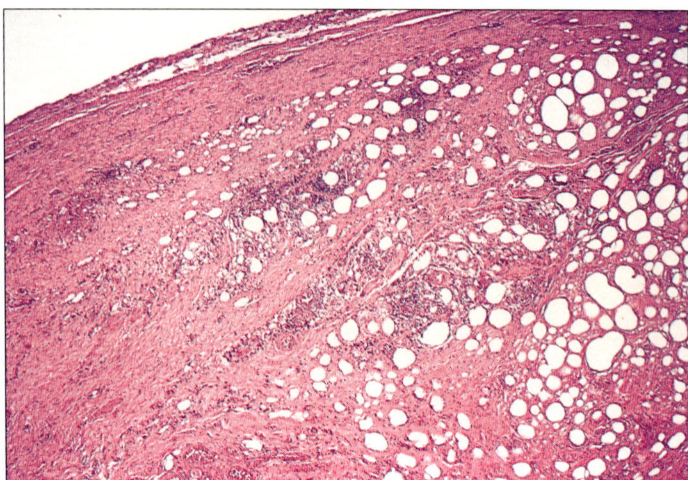

Figure 9.35 Sclerosing lipogranuloma of the genitalia. Large vacuoles that contained injected oily material are surrounded by dense fibrous tissue with chronic inflammatory cell infiltration.

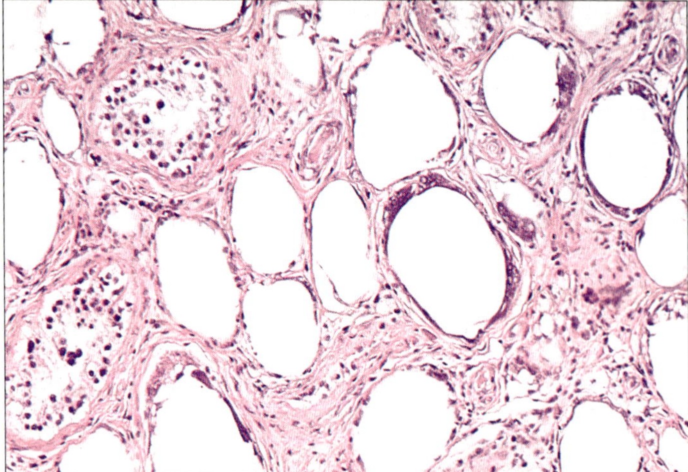

Figure 9.36 Sclerosing lipogranuloma of the genitalia. Large vacuoles that contained oily material are surrounded by dense fibrous tissue within the testis.

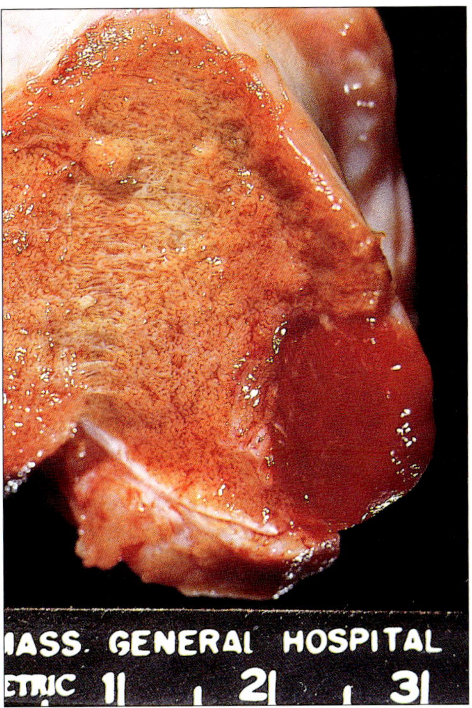

Figure 9.37 Splenic-gonadal fusion. A red, round nodule of splenic tissue occupies the lower pole of the testis.

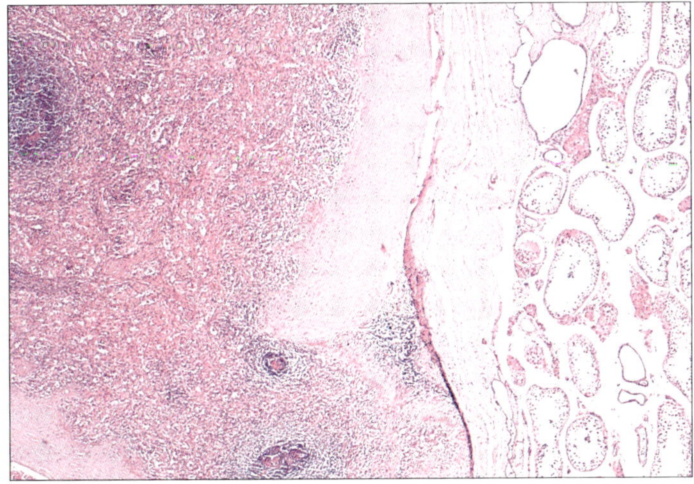

Figure 9.38 Splenic-gonadal fusion. Splenic tissue containing malpighian corpuscles lies to the right of testicular tissue, separated from it by the tunica albuginea.

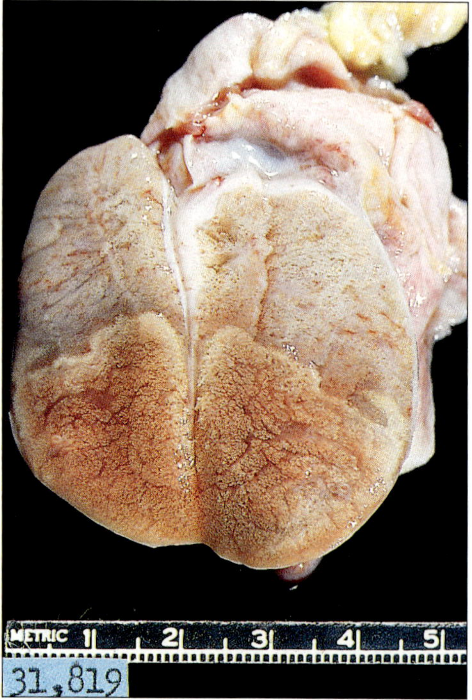

Figure 9.39 Infarct of testis. A pale infarct is bordered by a thin rim of reactive tissue.

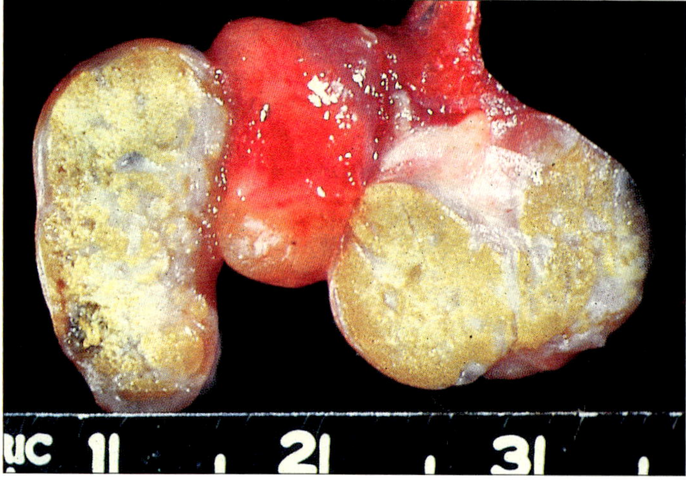

Figure 9.40 Infarct of testis. This old infarct, which simulated a neoplasm on clinical examination, has extensive yellow discoloration related to calcification.

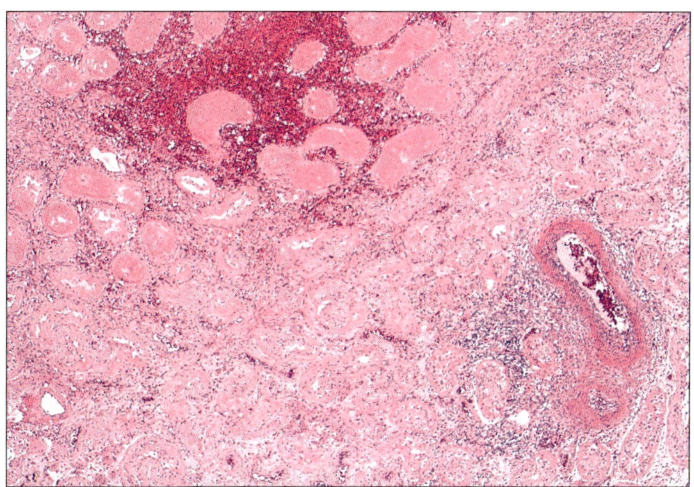

Figure 9.41 Infarct of testis. A focally hemorrhagic infarct in which the ghost remnants of tubules are visible was caused by necrotizing arteritis. An involved artery is present in the right portion of the photomicrograph.

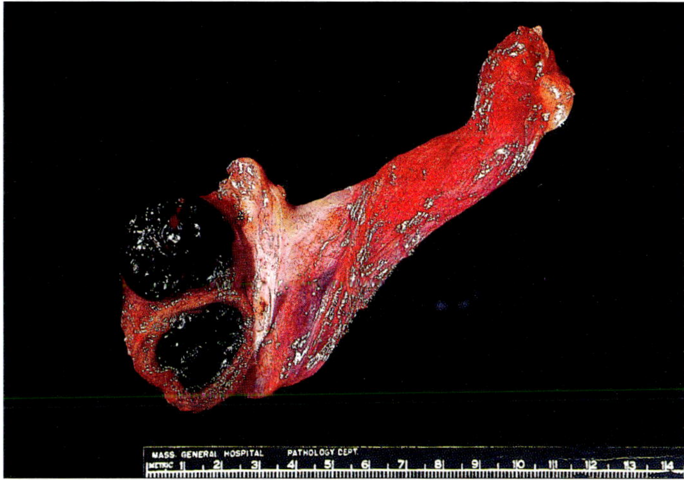

Figure 9.42 Hematoma of testis. A large, sharply circumscribed hematoma was caused by a localized necrotizing arteritis with rupture.

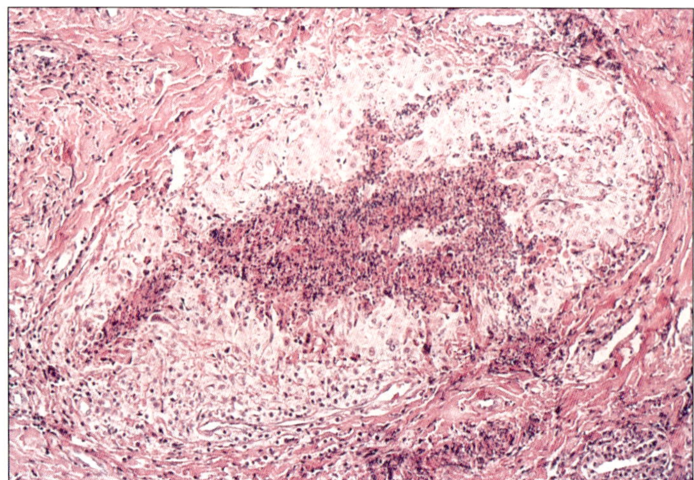

Figure 9.43 Sperm granuloma of epididymis. Closely packed basophilic sperm are surrounded by epithelioid cells, forming an oval nodule.

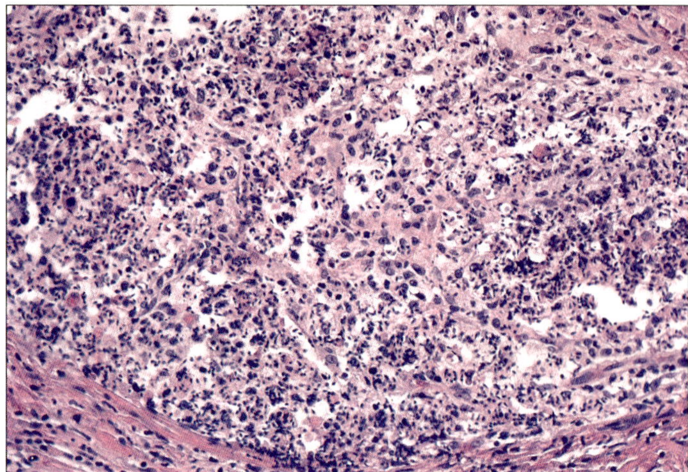

Figure 9.44 Sperm granuloma of epididymis. Basophilic sperm are admixed with epithelioid histiocytes.

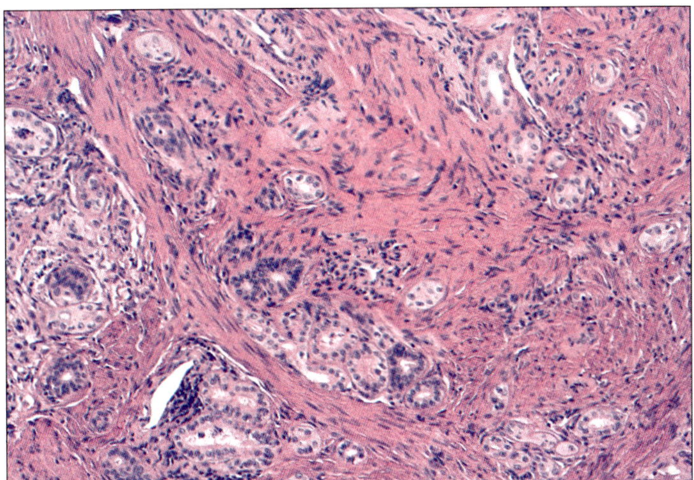

Figure 9.45 Vasitis nodosa. Small glandlike structures have infiltrated the muscularis of the vas deferens.

References

1. Dahl EV, Bahn RC. Aberrant adrenal cortical tissue near the testis in human infants. *Am J Pathol* 40:587–598, 1962.
2. Nelson AA. Accessory adrenal cortical tissue. *Arch Pathol* 27:955–965, 1939.
3. Rutgers JL, Young RH, Scully RE. The testicular 'tumor' of the adrenogenital syndrome: A report of five cases and review of the literature on testicular masses in patients with disorders of the adrenal glands. *Am J Surg Pathol* 12:503–513, 1988.
4. Price EB. Epidermoid cysts of the testis: A clinical and pathologic analysis of 69 cases from the testicular tumor registry. *J Urol* 102:708–713, 1969.
5. Shah KH, Maxted WC, Chun B. Epidermoid cysts of the testis: A report of three cases and analysis of 141 cases from the world literature. *Cancer* 47:577–582, 1981.
6. Van Niekerk WA. True hermaphroditism. *Pediatr Adolesc Endocrinol* 8:80–99, 1981.
7. Tesluk H, Blankenberg TA. Cystic dysplasia of testis. *Urology* 23:47–49, 1987.
8. Wegmann W, Illi O, Kummer-Vago M. Zystische Hodendysplasie mit ipsilateraler Nierenagenesie. *Schweiz Med Wochenschr* 114:144–148, 1984.
9. Nistal M. Regardera J, Paniagua R. Cystic dysplasia of the testis: Light and electron microscopic study of three cases. *Arch Pathol Lab Med* 108:579–583, 1984.
10. Honoré LH. Nonspecific peritesticular fibrosis manifested as testicular enlargement: Clinicopathological study of nine cases. *Arch Surg* 113:814–816, 1978.
11. Hourihane D O'B. Infected infarcts of the testis: A study of 18 cases preceded by pyogenic epididymo-orchitis. *J Clin Pathol* 23:668–675, 1970.
12. Gall EA. The histopathology of acute mumps orchitis. *Am J Pathol* 23:637–651, 1947.
13. Craighead JE, Mahoney EM, Carver DH, et al. Orchitis due to Coxsackie virus group B, types: Report of a case with isolation of virus from the testis. *N Engl J Med* 267:498–500, 1962.
14. Young RH, Scully RE. Miscellaneous neoplasms and non-neoplastic lesions. In: *Pathology of the Testis,* Talerman A, Roth LM, eds. *Contemporary Issues in Surgical Pathology*, vol 7. New York, Churchill Livingstone, 1986, chap 5.
15. Wechsler H, Westfall M, Lattimer JK. The earliest signs and symptoms in 127 male patients with genitourinary tuberculosis. *J Urol* 83:801–803, 1960.
16. Ferrie BG, Rundle JSH. Tuberculous epididymo-orchitis: A review of 20 cases. *Br J Urol* 55:437–439, 1983.
17. Grabstald H, Swan LL. Genitourinary lesions in leprosy, with special reference to the problem of atrophy of the testes. *JAMA* 149:1287–1291, 1952.
18. Menninger WC. Congenital syphilis of the testicle, with report of twelve autopsied cases. *Am J Syphilis* 12:221–234, 1928.

19. Morgan AD. Inflammatory lesions simulating malignancy. *Br J Urol* 36(suppl):95–102, 1964.

20. Spjut H, Thorpe J. Granulomatous orchitis. *Am J Clin Pathol* 26:136–145, 1956.

21. Amenta PS, Gonick P, Katz SM. Sarcoidosis of testis and epididymis. *Urology* 17:616–617, 1981.

22. McClure J. Malakoplakia. *J Pathol* 140:275–330, 1983.

23. McClure J. Malakoplakia of the testis and its relationship to granulomatous orchitis. *J Clin Pathol* 33:670–678, 1980.

24. Benisch B, Peison B, Sobel HJ, Marquet E. Fibrous mesotheliomas (pseudofibroma) of the scrotal sac: A light and ultrastructural study. *Cancer* 47:731–735, 1981.

25. Lowenthal SB, Goldstein AMB, Terry R. Cholesterol granuloma of tunica vaginalis simulating testicular tumor. *Urology* 18:89–90, 1981.

26. Oertel YC, Johnson FB. Sclerosing lipogranuloma of male genitalia: Review of 23 cases. *Arch Pathol Lab Med* 101:321–326, 1977.

27. Putschar WG, Manion WC. Splenic-gonadal fusion. *Am J Pathol* 32:15–33, 1956.

28. Pendse AK, Mathur PN, Sharma MM, Gupta OP. Splenic-gonadal fusion. *Br J Surg* 62:624–628, 1975.

29. Walter MM, Trulock TS, Finnerty DP, Woodard J. Splenic gonadal fusion. *Urology* 32:521–524, 1988.

30. Skoglund RW, McRoberts JW, Ragde H. Torsion of the spermatic cord: A review of the literature and an analysis of 70 new cases. *J Urol* 104:604–607, 1970.

31. Shurbaji MS, Epstein JI. Testicular vasculitis: Implications for systemic disease. *Hum Pathol* 19:186–189, 1988.

32. Dahl EV, Baggenstoss AH, DeWeerd JH. Testicular lesions of periarteritis nodosa with special reference to diagnosis. *Am J Med* 28:222–228, 1960.

33. Friedman NB, Garske GL. Inflammatory reactions involving sperm and the seminiferous tubules: Extravasation, spermatic granulomas and granulomatous orchitis. *J Urol* 62:363–374, 1949.

34. Glassy FJ, Mostofi FK. Spermatic granulomas of the epididymis. *Am J Clin Pathol* 26:1303–1313, 1956.

35. Benjamin JA, Robertson TD, Cheetham JG. Vasitis nodosa: A new clinical entity simulating tuberculosis of the vas deferens. *J Urol* 49:575–582, 1943.

36. Civantos F, Lubin J, Rywlin AM. Vasitis nodosa. *Arch Pathol* 94:355–361, 1972.

37. Kovi J, Agbata A. Benign neural invasion in vasitis nodosa. *JAMA* 228:1519, 1974.

Index

Numbers in **boldface** refer to pages on which illustrations appear.

ACTH. *See* Adrenocorticotropic hormone
Acute lymphoblastic leukemia, 153, **158**
Adenocarcinoma
  metastatic, of prostate, 153, **158–159**
  papillary. *See* Papillary adenocarcinoma
Adenoma
  papillary, of rete testis, 165, **177–179**
  Sertoli cell, 140, **144, 148–149**
Adenomatoid tumor, 163–164, **169–171**
Adrenocortical rest, 189, **199–200**
Adrenocorticotropic hormone (ACTH), 190
Adrenogenital syndrome (AGS), testicular tumor of, 189–191, **201–202**
Adult-type granulosa cell tumor, 106–107, **127–128**
AFP stain. 40, 45, **61**
Alkaline phosphatase, placental-like, 12–13, 91
Androgen insensitivity syndrome, 140–141, **144–149**
  hamartomas in, 141, **147–148**
  intratubular germ cell neoplasia in cases of, 141
  Leydig cells in, 140, **144–146**
  ovarian stroma in, 140, **144–146**
  seminoma in, 141, **147, 149**
  Sertoli cell adenoma in, 140, **144, 148–149**
Androstenedione, 190
Argentaffin granules, in carcinoid tumor, 43, **69**
Arteritis, 197
Artifactual pseudoinvasion of blood vessels, 4, **6**
Atypical epithelial cells, in epididymis, 166, **180**

Bacterial orchitis, 192
Bilateral germ cell tumors, 10
Brenner tumor, 165
Burkitt's lymphoma, 152

Call-Exner bodies, 105–106, 108, **127, 133**
Carcinoid tumor, 42–43, **69–70**
  metastatic to testis, 153
Carcinoma
  embryonal. *See* Embryonal carcinoma
  metastatic, 153–154
  of rete testis, 165, **177–179**
Charcot-Böttcher filament bundles, 106, 138
Chemotherapy
  germ cell tumors after, 46–47, **81–83**
Cholesterol granuloma, 196
Choriocarcinoma, 40–41, **61–62**
  as component of mixed germ cell tumor, 44, **75**
  cytotrophoblast cells in, 40, **62**
  intermediate trophoblast cells in, 41, **62–64**
  Leydig cell hyperplasia and, 41, **63**
  syncytiotrophoblast cells in, 41, **62**
Choriocarcinoma-like lesion, after chemotherapy, 41, 47
Classification of testicular tumors, 1–3
Clear cell papillary adenocarcinoma, of testis, 164–165, **175–176**
Coxsackie B virus, 192
Cryptorchidism, 10, 139, 141
  associated with intratubular germ cell neoplasia, 91
Cushing's disease, 190
Cyst, 191, **203**
  epidermoid, 191, **203**
  müllerian, 141
  wolffian, 141
Cystadenoma, papillary. *See* Papillary cystadenoma
Cystic dysplasia, 191, **204**
Cytokeratin staining

of embryonal carcinoma for, 38, **52**
of seminoma for, 12
of yolk sac tumor for, 40

Diethylstilbestrol, 165
Diffuse embryoma, 45, **77–79**
Dysgenetic male pseudohermaphroditism, 137–138
Dysplasia, cystic, 191, **204**

Embryoid bodies, 41, **64–65**
Embryoma, diffuse, 45, **77–79**
Embryonal carcinoma, 5, 10, 37–38, **48–52**
as component of mixed germ cell tumor, 5, 44–45, **73–74, 76**
cytokeratins in, 38, 52
in diffuse embryoma, 45, **77–78**
glandular pattern, 37, **49**
granulomas in, 38
hematogenous metastasis of, 38, **52**
immunohistochemistry of, 38, **52**
with immature mesenchyme, 38, **51**
intratubular, 92, **96–97**
in mixed germ cell tumor, 44–45, **72–74, 76**
papillary pattern, 37, **50**
solid pattern, 37, **49**
tubular pattern, **37**
with syncytiotrophoblast cells, 37–38, **51**
vascular invasion by, **6**
Endodermal sinus tumor. *See* Yolk sac tumor
Endometrioid adenocarcinoma, 164
Endometriosis, paratesticular, 165, **176**
Epidermoid cyst, 191, **203**
Epididymis
adenomatoid tumor of, 163, **169–171**
adrenocortical rest in, 189, **200**
atypical epithelial cells in, 166, **180**
papillary adenocarcinoma of, 166, **179–180**
papillary cystadenoma, 166, **179**
retinal anlage tumor of, 167, **181–183**
sperm granuloma of, 197, **220**
Epididymo-orchitis, tuberculous, **207–208**
Epithelial cells, atypical, in epididymis, **180**
Escherichia coli, 195
Evaluation of testicular tumors, 4–5
Exophthalmos, in patients with seminoma, 10

Factor VIII–related antigen, 4
α-Fetoprotein (AFP) stain, 40, 45, **61**
Ferritin, staining for in intratubular germ cell neoplasia, 91
Fibroma, 168, **184**
Fibromatous periorchitis, 195, **215**
Fibrosarcoma, **185**
Fibrous histiocytoma, 168
Fibrous pseudotumor, 195, **215**

Germ cell neoplasia, intratubular. *See* Intratubular germ cell neoplasia
Germ cell–sex cord–stromal tumor, unclassified, 139, **144**
Germ cell tumor
metastatic, retroperitoneal, after chemotherapy, **81–83**
mixed, 4–5, 44–46, **71–73**
nonseminomatous, 11, 37–47, **48–83**
occult, 46, **79–81**
retrogressed, **80–81**
Germinoma, 139
Glial fibrillary acidic protein staining, of primitive neuroectodermal tumor, 43
Gonadal dysgenesis, mixed, 137–139, **142–143**
Gonadoblastoma, 138–140, **142–143**
Granuloma, 11
cholesterol, 196
sperm, 197, **220**
Granulomatous orchitis, 193–194, **207–210**
Granulosa cell tumor
adult-type, 106–107, **127–128**
juvenile-type, 107, **128–131**
in patients with mixed gonadal dysgenesis, 139
Grimelius staining, of carcinoid tumor, 43

Gumma, 193, **208–209**
Gynecomastia, 10, 40, 108

Hamartoma, in androgen insensitivity syndrome, 141, **147–148**
  melanotic. *See* Retinal anlage tumor
Hemangioendothelioma, **184**
Hemangioma, 167–168, **184**
Hematoma, 197, **219**
Hermaphroditism
  true, 139–140
  pseudo-, dysgenetic male, 137–138
Histiocytoma, fibrous, 168
Histological classification of tumors, 1–3
Hodgkin's disease, 152
Human chorionic gonadotropin, 10, 12, **27,** 38, 41
21-Hydroxylase deficiency, 189–190
17-Hydroxyprogesterone, 190
Hyperplasia, Leydig cell, 41, **63**

Idiopathic granulomatous orchitis, 193–194, **209–210**
  epithelioid histiocytes in, 194, **210**
  Langhans' giant cells in, 194, **210**
Incidence of germ cell tumors, 9
Infarct, 197, **218–219**
Infectious granulomatous orchitis
  lepromatous, 193
  syphilitic, 193, **208–209**
  tuberculous, 193, **207–208**
Infertility, associated with intratubular germ cell neoplasia, 90–91
Intersexual disorder, 137–141, **142–149**
Intratubular embryonal carcinoma, 92, **96–97**
Intratubular germ cell neoplasia, 89–93, **94–98**
  classification of, 89
  unclassified, 89–92, **94–95, 98,** 141
  unclassified with extratubular infiltration, 92, **98**
Intratubular seminoma, 92, **95–97**
Intratubular spermatocytic seminoma, 92, **97**
Intratubular yolk sac tumor, 93
Intravascular tumor, **6**

Juvenile granulosa cell tumor, 107, **128–132**
  in patients with mixed gonadal dysgenesis, 139

17-Ketosteroids, in patients with adrenogenital syndrome, 190

Langhans'-type giant cells, in idiopathic granulomatous orchitis, 194, **210**
Langhans'-type giant cells, in seminoma, 11, **22**
Large cell calcifying Sertoli cell tumor, 105–106, **122–125**
Large cell Sertoli cell tumor, 104, **126**
Leiomyoma, 167
Leiomyosarcoma, 168
Leprosy, 193
Leukemia, acute lymphoblastic, 153, **158**
Leydig cell hyperplasia, in association with choriocarcinoma, 41, **63**
Leydig cell tumor, 101–104, **110–117**
  benign vs malignant, 102
  crystals of Reinke in, 102, **115**
  in androgen insensitivity syndrome, 141
  psammoma bodies in, 102, **116**
  spindle cells in, 102, **115**
Lipogranuloma, sclerosing, 196, **216**
Lipoma, 168
Liposarcoma, 168
Lung cancer, metastatic to testis, 153
Lymphoma, malignant, 151–152, **155–157**

Malakoplakia, 194–195, **211–214**
  differential diagnosis with Leydig cell tumor, 103
Malaria, 197
Malignant fibrous histocytoma, 168
Malignant lymphoma. *See* Lymphoma, malignant
Malignant mesothelioma. *See* Mesothelioma, malignant

Masson-Fontana staining of carcinoid tumor, 43, **70**
Melanoma, malignant, metastatic, 153, **159–160**
Melanotic hamartoma, progonoma, neuroectodermal tumor. *See* Retinal anlage tumor
Mesothelioma, malignant, of tunica vaginalis, 164–166, **172–174**
Metastatic tumor, from testis, after chemotherapy, 46–47, **81–83**
Metastatic tumor, from testis, choriocarcinoma-like lesion in, 41, 47
Metastatic tumor, from testis, malignant change in, 47
Metastatic tumor to testis, 153–154, **159–160**
Michaelis-Gutmann bodies, 195, **213–214**
Micrognathia, 196
Mixed germ cell tumor, 44–46, **71–79**
  with choriocarcinoma, 44, **75**
  criteria for diagnosis of, 45
  diffuse embryoma in, 45, **77–79**
  quantitation of elements, 4–5
  with embryonal carcinoma, 44–45, **72–74,** 76
  with seminoma, 44, **72–75**
  with teratoma, 44–45, **72–73, 75**
  with yolk sac tumor, 45, **76**
Mixed gonadal dysgenesis, 137–139, **142–143**
Mucinous cystadenocarcinoma, 164
Mucinous cystadenoma, 164
Müllerian cyst, 141
Mumps orchitis, 192–193, **206**
Multiple myeloma, 152–153

Nelson's syndrome, 190
Neuroectodermal tumor
  melanotic. *See* Retinal anlage tumor
  primitive, 43–44, **70–71**
Neurofibroma, 168
  paratesticular, **183**
Neuron specific enolase, staining of seminoma, 12
Nodular periorchitis, 195, **215**
Nodular precocious maturation, 192, **205**
Nodule, Sertoli cell, 105, **121–122**
Nonneoplastic lesions, 189–198, **199–221**
Nonseminomatous germ cell tumors, 37–47, **48–83**

Occult germ cell tumor, 46
  intratubular germ cell neoplasia in patient with, 46, **90**
  mature teratoma as, 46, **80**
  retrogressed, 46, **80–81**
  seminoma as, 46, **79**
Orchitis
  bacterial, 192
  granulomatous, 193–194, **207–210**
    idiopathic, 193–194, **209–210**
    infectious, 193, **207–209**
  mumps, 192–193, **206**
  tuberculous epididymo-, 193, **207–208**
  viral, 152, 192–193, **206–207**
Osteosarcoma, 168
Ovarian-type tumor, 164–165, **174–176**
Ovotestes, 139

Papillary adenocarcinoma, clear cell
  of epididymis, 166, **180**
  of testis, 165, **175–176**
Papillary adenoma, of rete testis, 165, **177–179**
Papillary cystadenoma of epididymis, 166, **179**
Periarteritis nodosa, 197
Periorchitis
  fibromatous, 195, **215**
Peutz-Jeghers syndrome, 105, **126**
Phosphatase, placental-like alkaline, 12–13, 91
  staining for in embryonal carcinoma, 38
  staining for in intratubular germ cell neoplasia, 91
  staining for in seminoma, 12
  staining for in yolk sac tumor, 40
Placental lactogen (hPL), 41, **64**
Placental site trophoblastic tumor, 41, **63–64**
Plasmacytoma, 152–153, **157**

Polyembryoma, 41, **64–65**
Precocious maturation, nodular, 192, **205**
Primitive neuroectodermal tumor, 43–44, **70–71**
Progonoma, melanotic. *See* Retinal anlage tumor
Prostate, adenocarcinoma of, metastatic, 153, **158–159**
  confusion with Leydig cell tumor, 103
Pseudohermaphroditism, dysgenetic male, 137–138
Pseudohyperplasia, of rete testis, **178**
Pseudoinvasion of blood vessels, artifactual, 4, **6**
Pseudotumor, fibrous, 195, **215**

Rete testis
  adenocarcinoma of, 165–166, **177–179**
  adenoma, 165
  papillary adenoma of, 165, **177**
  pseudohyperplasia of, 166, **178**
Retinal anlage tumor, 167, **181–183**
Retrogressed germ cell tumor, 46, **80–81**
Rhabdomyosarcoma
  arising in teratoma, **69**
  intratesticular, 168
  paratesticular, 168
  with spermatocytic seminoma, 12, **31–32**
Rosettes, in primitive neuroectodermal tumor, 43, **71**

Sarcoidosis, 194
Sarcoma
  with spermatocytic seminoma, 13, **31**
  of testis, 168, 185
Scar
  in cases of occult germ cell tumor, 46, **80–81, 83**
  in seminoma, 11, **23**
  in metastatic tumor after chemotherapy, 46, **81**
Schiller-Duval bodies, 39, **53–54**
Sclerosing lipogranuloma, 196, **216**
Seminoma, **6,** 9–12, **14–26,** 141, 152
  anaplastic, 9–10
  in androgen insensitivity syndrome, **147, 149**
  artifact due to improper fixation, 11, **25**
  cords in, 10, 18
  frequency of, 10
  gland-like spaces in, 10, **19**
  glycogen granules in, 11, **24**
  granulomatous reaction in, 11, **22**
  gross appearance of, 10, **14–16**
  immunohistochemistry of, 12, **27**
  intratubular, 92, **95–97**
  with lymphoid follicles, 11, **21**
  in androgen insensitivity syndrome, 141, **149**
  in mixed germ cell tumor, **73–75**
  mitotic figures in, 9–11, **24**
  necrosis in, 11, **16, 23**
  nests in, 10, **17–18**
  occult, 46, **79**
  pagetoid spread to rete testis, 11, **20**
  scar in, 11, **23**
  solid tubules in, 10–11, **20**
  spermatocytic, 10, 12–13, **28–32, 97,** 152
    intratubular, **30, 97**
    with nonspecific sarcoma, 13, **31**
    with rhabdomyosarcoma, 13, **31–32**
  syncytiophoblast giant cells in, 11, **26–27**
  typical, 9–10
Serous carcinoma, 164
Serous papillary cystadenoma of borderline malignancy, 164–165, **174–175**
Sertoli cell nodule in cryptorchid testis, 105, **121–122**
Sertoli cell tumor, 104–106, **117–126**
  adenoma, 140, **144, 148–149**
  in androgen insensitivity syndrome, 140, **144, 148–149**
  large cell calcifying, 105–106, **122–126**
  metastatic to bone, **121**
Sex cord–stromal tumors, 101–109, **110–134**

unclassified, 108–109, **132–134**
Soft tissue tumors, 167–168, **183–185**
Spermatocytic seminoma, 12–13, **28–32, 97,** 152
intratubular, 13, **30,** 92, **97**
metastasis of, 13
with nonspecific sarcoma, 13, **31**
with rhabdomyosarcoma, 13, **31–32**
Sperm granuloma, of epididymis, 197, **220**
Splenic-gonadal fusion, 196–197, **217**
Staging of testicular tumors, 3–4
Streak testes, 137–138
Synctiotrophoblast giant cells, in seminoma, 10–11, **26–27**
Syphilis, 193, **208–209**
gumma of testis, **208–209**

Teratoma, 41–42, **66–69**
carcinoid tumor associated with, 43
choriocarcinoma and, **75**
immature, 42, **68**
malignant transformation of, 42, **69**
mature, 42, 47, **66–67, 82–83**
occult, **80**
in mixed germ cell tumor, **72–73, 75**
metastatic, **82–83**
rhabdomyosarcoma arising in, 42, **69**
seminoma and, **75**
Testicular feminization. *See* Androgen insensitivity syndrome
Testicular "tumor" of adrenogenital syndrome, 189–191, **201–202**
TNM staging. *See* Tumor node metastasis staging
Trophoblastic tumor, placental site, 41, **63–64**
Tuberculosis, 193, **207–208**
epididymo-orchitis, **207–208**
Tumor lymph node metastasis (TNM) staging, 3–4
Tunica albuginea
adenomatoid tumor of, 163, **169**
fibroma of, **184**
Tunica vaginalis
calcification of, 196
mesothelioma of, 164–166, **172–174**

Ulex europaeus lectin antigens, 4
Undescended testes. *See* Cryptorchidism

Vascular invasion, by embryonal carcinoma, 4, **6**
Vasitis nodosa, 198, **221**
Vimentin, staining of seminoma for, 12, **27**
Viral orchitis, 152, 192–193
interstitial hemorrhage in, 192–193, **206**
mumps, 192–193, **206**
von Hansemann cells, 103, 195, **211–212**
von Hippel–Lindau disease, 166, **179**
von Kossa stain, 195, **214**

Wolffian cyst, 141
World Health Organization classification, 1–3

Yolk sac tumor, 38–40, 45, **53–60, 76**
α-fetoprotein in, 40, **61**
as component of mixed germ cell tumor, 44–45, **76**
in children, 38–39, **53**
clear cytoplasm, in cells of, 40, **60**
in diffuse embryoma, 45, **77–78**
embryonal carcinoma with, 76
festoon pattern, **56**
glandular pattern, 39, **59**
gross appearance of, 39, **53**
hepatocyte-like cells in, 39, 58
hyaline globules in, 40, **55, 59**
immunohistochemistry of, 40, **61**
liposarcoma mimicry, 39, **55**
macrocystic pattern, 39
microcystic pattern, 39, **54**
mucinous glands in, 39, **58**
myxoid stroma, **60**
papillary pattern, 39, **56**
parietal pattern, 39, **57**
polyvesicular pattern, 39, **57**
reticular pattern, 39, **53**
Schiller-Duval bodies in, 39, **53–54**
solid pattern, 39, **55, 60**
stroma, appearance of, 40
vacuolated cells in, 39, **55**